Basic Guide to
Anatomy and Physiology
for Dental Care Professionals

D1500834

For Mum and Dad,
Penny and Ian, and Tony and Margaret – love always.

BASIC GUIDE TO ANATOMY AND PHYSIOLOGY FOR DENTAL CARE PROFESSIONALS

Carole Hollins

Dental Surgeon and Training Course Facilitator, Stoke-on-Trent, UK
Chairman, NEBDN, Fleetwood, UK

⊛WILEY-BLACKWELL

A John Wiley & Sons, Ltd., Publication

This edition first published 2012
© 2012 by John Wiley & Sons, Ltd.

Wiley-Blackwell is an imprint of John Wiley & Sons, formed by the merger of Wiley's global
Scientific, Technical and Medical business with Blackwell Publishing.

Registered office: John Wiley & Sons, Ltd, The Atrium, Southern Gate, Chichester, West Sussex,
PO19 8SQ, UK

Editorial offices: 9600 Garsington Road, Oxford, OX4 2DQ, UK
The Atrium, Southern Gate, Chichester, West Sussex, PO19 8SQ, UK
2121 State Avenue, Ames, Iowa 50014-8300, USA

For details of our global editorial offices, for customer services and for information about how to
apply for permission to reuse the copyright material in this book please see our website at
www.wiley.com/wiley-blackwell.

Library of Congress Cataloging-in-Publication Data
Hollins, Carole.
  Basic guide to anatomy and physiology for dental care professionals / Carole Hollins.
    p. ; cm.
  Includes bibliographical references and index.
  ISBN 978-0-470-65611-2 (pbk. : alk. paper)
  I. Title.
  [DNLM: 1. Anatomy. 2. Physiological Phenomena. 3. Stomatognathic System–anatomy &
histology. QS 4]
  612–dc23

                                                                              2012011413

A catalogue record for this book is available from the British Library.

Wiley also publishes its books in a variety of electronic formats. Some content that appears in
print may not be available in electronic books.

Cover image: courtesy of Carole Hollins
Cover design by Workhaus

Set in 10/12.5pt Sabon by Aptara® Inc., New Delhi, India
Printed and bound in Malaysia by Vivar Printing Sdn Bhd

1 2012

Contents

How to use this book

This book is one of the 'Basic Guide' series published by Wiley-Blackwell.

'Dental Care Professional' (DCP) is the title given to all members of the oral health care team besides the dentist, who are involved in some way in the care and/or treatment of the patient. The title includes all of the following:

- Dental nurses, including those with extended duties
- Dental hygienists
- Dental therapists
- Clinical dental technicians

Each category of registerable members has a specific role to play in assisting the patient to achieve and maintain a good standard of oral health. Without exception, however, they all need to have an adequate level of knowledge and understanding in the key areas of anatomy and physiology, in relation to dentistry and dental treatment, to be able to carry out that role.

This book has been written with the aim of giving that underpinning knowledge to the readership, whether they are clinical dental technicians providing a set of full dentures to the patient without prescription from the dentist, or a dental nurse assisting the dentist at the chair side.

The depth of knowledge required to be understood in each chapter will vary between the DCP groups, in line with their specific curricular requirements, and all readers are advised to ensure that they follow the text in line with those requirements. However, it is hoped that the text is written in such a way as to generate a thirst for further knowledge among at least some of the readership.

The basics of biology are covered in the first chapter, along with information on disease processes and anatomical nomenclature. The four main body systems are then covered in the following chapters, including dentally relevant medical conditions of those systems, along with information on the types of medication that sufferers are likely to be prescribed. It is hoped that the inclusion of this information will enable readers to better understand the significance of various medical conditions and medications that patients often record in their medical histories.

Before moving on to the chapters covering the specialised areas of the oral cavity that are of major interest to DCPs, a chapter is included that covers the basics of oral embryology – this is to help the readers in their understanding not only of the early development of the relevant oral structures, but also to give an insight into how some dental conditions develop. Again, the depth of knowledge of interest to each group will vary throughout the text.

The final chapters cover the anatomy of the skull, and the structure and function of teeth, the periodontium and the salivary glands. The information provided should enable the readers to better understand the fine workings of these oral structures, and the disease processes that can affect them.

Overall, it is hoped that the text content provides the reader with a greater understanding of the workings of the human body in relation to oral and general health, as well as oral and general disease. The diagrams used are coloured for clarity, so that structures can be more easily visualised.

Chapter 1

Basic biology – overview

It is very important for all dental care professionals (DCPs) to have a good underpinning knowledge of the normal structure and function of the human body, and especially of their specialised area – the oral cavity and its surroundings.

This knowledge is essential when trying to understand the subjects of human health, the processes involved in the onset of human disease and the methods available to prevent disease or to treat it when already present.

DEFINITIONS

The scientific discipline that deals with the life processes of living organisms is called **biology**, and the specific area for this text is **human biology**.

The particular study of the structures of the human body and their relationships to one another is called **human anatomy**, and the study of how the body actually functions is called **human physiology**.

The subject of anatomy covers not only the gross structure of the human body – muscles, bones, organs, and so on – but also the equally important microscopic structures of the cells and tissues themselves that make up these gross structures.

The study of the microscopic structure and function of cells, and the tissues that they form, is called **histology**.

CELL BIOLOGY

The structures and functions of the human body as a living organism work in a similar way to those of a complicated machine that follows the laws of both chemistry and physics for its operation.

At the most basic level, all the structures of the body are made up of atoms arranged in specific ways that identify them as **chemical elements,** such as

Basic Guide to Anatomy and Physiology for Dental Care Professionals, First Edition. Carole Hollins.
© 2012 John Wiley & Sons, Ltd. Published 2012 by John Wiley & Sons, Ltd.

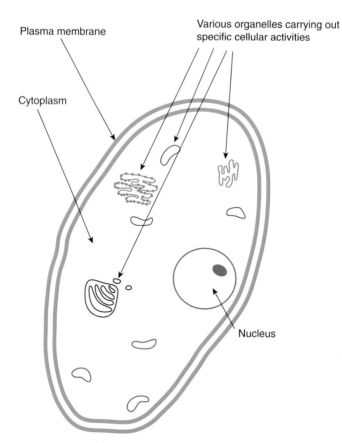

Plasma membrane

Various organelles carrying out specific cellular activities

Cytoplasm

Nucleus

Figure 1.1 Basic structure of the cell.

oxygen, hydrogen and carbon. When these different elements combine together they form **molecules,** such as water and carbon dioxide.

When the molecules themselves combine together in many different ways, they form the basic unit of any living organism – **the cell**.

The microscopic structure of a basic cell is shown in Figure 1.1 and is composed of the following:

- **Plasma membrane** – the outer border of the cell itself that holds all of the contents together
- **Cytoplasm** – the inner fluid of the cell, where all of the internal structures are suspended
- **Organelles** – specialised structures within the cell, each with their own specific function, such as waste disposal, food production and energy conversion
- **Nucleus** – the main organelle of all body cells (except red blood cells) that acts as the control centre of the cell by directing the various actions of all

of the other organelles, such as energy conversion, growth, food production and waste disposal

It is within the nucleus that the genetic code is stored (usually referred to just as 'DNA' by the lay public), so the nucleus controls all of the cell functions and directs its activities.

Most cells are specialised in their actions and perform certain functions within the body. When they are grouped together to carry out these particular functions, they are called **tissues**.

The main types of tissue found in the body are:

- **Muscle tissue** – generate forces and produce motion; can be attached to bones to allow the movement of limbs (**skeletal muscle**), or enclose hollow cavities (**smooth muscle**) so that they can squeeze around the cavity and remove its contents (such as in the digestive system), or be a third specialised type found only in the heart and called **cardiac muscle**
- **Nervous tissue** – initiate and carry electrical impulses along their length to distant areas of the body to effect muscle contractions, gland secretions, and so on
- **Epithelial tissue** – form the outer layer of the body, as skin, or surround specific groups of tissues to form organs, or line hollow structures within the body, and also separate various areas from each other to avoid the uncontrolled movement of micro-organisms throughout the body
- **Connective tissue** – connect various parts of the body together to give anchorage and support, such as the connection together of various bones in a joint by tendons and ligaments
- **Blood and lymph tissue** – are often classed as types of connective tissue, but are unique in existing as cells within a fluid, rather than being a continuous mass of cells like other connective tissues

When several different groups of tissues exist together and carry out a particular function (or functions) they form an **organ**, such as the heart, the liver, the spleen, and so on.

Organs that have related functions then form integral parts of **body systems**, such as the digestive system, the respiratory system, and so on.

These will be summarised later.

BASIC TISSUES

The four main basic tissue types will be covered in greater depth to help give a greater understanding of their structure and functions within the oral cavity.

Although separated out in the previous list, blood and lymph will be grouped together with the other connective tissues.

Muscle tissue

This tissue develops from the mesoderm layer of the early embryo, once the developing inner cell cluster has organised into a flat disc at around 3 weeks after fertilisation (see Chapter 6).

All muscle tissue acts by being innervated by the electrical impulses transmitted by nerve cells, causing the contraction (shortening) of the muscle tissue itself. The resultant action produced depends on the surrounding structures that the muscle tissue is connected to.

Muscle tissue can be classified into three groups, depending on their structure, their function and which part of the nervous system activates them:

- Skeletal muscle
- Smooth muscle
- Cardiac muscle

Skeletal muscle has the following characteristics:

- Connected at one or both ends to bones by tendons and ligaments
- Considered as **voluntary muscle** because they are innervated by somatic nerves (a type of motor nerve), so their contraction can be consciously controlled to produce the voluntary movement of parts of the musculoskeletal system
- Cannot carry out prolonged contraction without tiring, and requiring a rest period
- Microscopically, they are composed of bundles of cell fibres running the length of the tissue, and appear to be striped or **striated**
- Dentally relevant skeletal muscles include the following:
  - Muscles of mastication
  - Muscles of facial expression
  - The tongue
  - Suprahyoid muscles
  - Muscles of the pharynx

Smooth muscle has the following characteristics:

- Located in the walls of blood vessels, in hollow organs such as parts of the digestive system, and in glands
- Considered as **involuntary muscle** because they are innervated by the autonomic nervous system, so their actions cannot be consciously controlled
- Do not tire, as skeletal muscle does
- Microscopically, they are composed of sheets of elongated cells bound in connective tissue, with no striations
- The sheets of cells can run both lengthways and in a circular fashion, so their contraction produces a wave of squeeze-like actions along vessels or in organs and glands

- Unlike skeletal muscle, smooth muscles do not tend to be individually named
- Dentally relevant locations of smooth muscle are:
  - All blood vessels
  - Salivary glands
  - Various areas of the oral cavity, beneath other structures

Cardiac muscle has the following characteristics:

- Specialised type of **striated** muscle that occurs in the wall of the heart only
- Considered as **involuntary muscle** because it is innervated by the autonomic nervous system, and cannot be consciously controlled
- Does not tire, otherwise the heart would stop beating and death would occur
- Rate of contraction can be increased or decreased depending on the needs of the body for its supply of oxygenated blood
- Microscopically, the rod-shaped cells run together in a three-dimensional pattern, and interconnect with each other in a grid system so that innervation occurs in a controlled wave across the surface of the heart, producing the heart beat

The microscopic appearance of the three muscle types are illustrated in Figure 1.2.

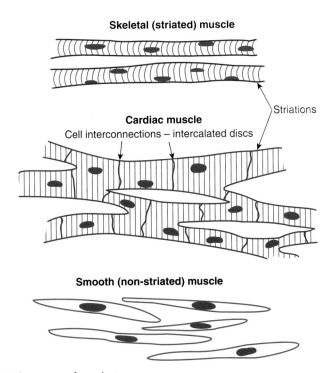

Figure 1.2 Three types of muscle tissue.

Nervous tissue

This tissue develops from the outer layer of cells of the early embryo, the ectoderm and its specialised sub-layer the neuroectoderm.

The specialised sensory cells of the eyes, the nose, the ears and the taste buds of the tongue are all part of the nervous system, but the basic nerve cell is the **neurone.**

All neurones function by carrying electrical impulses around the entire body. The electrical impulses can only travel in one direction, so one set of nerve cells transmits impulses from the body to the brain, and another set transmits impulses from the brain to the body.

The neurones of each set of nerve type are arranged in long chains through-out the length of each nerve, interconnecting one with the next neurone in the chain.

Within the brain itself are specialised neurones and their support cells, which are discussed in more detail in Chapter 5.

Nervous tissue making up the peripheral nervous system (that outside the brain and spinal cord) can be simply classified into two groups, depending on the direction of travel of the electrical impulses that they transmit:

- **Sensory nerves** –carry information from the body to the brain, for analysis and interpretation by the specialised cells within
- **Motor nerves** –transmit action impulses from the brain to various areas of the body, and can be sub-divided further as follows:
  - **Somatic nerves** – carry impulses to the musculoskeletal system
  - **Autonomic nerves** – carry impulses to blood vessels, organs and glands

A typical neurone is made up of three sections, the cell body and two types of cytoplasmic projection, and is illustrated in Figure 1.3.

The cell body itself is the support structure for the neurone, and contains all of the usual cellular contents: a nucleus, various organelles, and so on.

Extending from the cell body are various small projections called **dendrites,** which receive the electrical impulses from the previous neurone and pass them towards the cell body. The cell body itself is not involved in the impulse trans-mission, and the electrical activity continues on to the other cytoplasmic pro-jection, the **axon.**

The axon is a much longer projection than the dendrites and is surrounded by its own cell membrane, which is responsible for the continued impulse transmission along the neurone, away from the cell body.

The method of electrical impulse transmission is explained in Chapter 5.

In many nerves throughout the body, the axon also has a fatty covering along its length, interrupted periodically by tiny points of non-coverage called **nodes of Ranvier.**

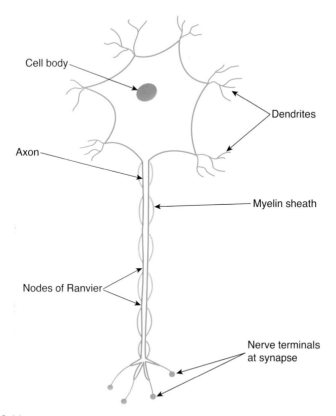

Figure 1.3 Neurone.

In these nerves, the electrical impulse is able to leap-frog along the axon by jumping from node to node, and in this way the impulse is transmitted far more quickly than would otherwise be possible.

The point at which one neurone connects with another, or with the tissue that it is to innervate, is called the **synapse**. At this point, the electrical impulse is further transmitted by chemicals called **neurotransmitters**.

Epithelial tissue

This tissue develops from all three layers of cells in the early embryo – the ectoderm, the mesoderm and the endoderm – and the layer of origin determines the final tissue and its function in the body.

So, a simple overview is as follows:

- **Ectoderm origin** – develop into the skin and the inner linings of hollow body organs and systems, such as the digestive tract and the lungs
- **Mesoderm origin** – develop into the epithelial sheaths surrounding the heart, the lungs and the abdominal cavity, and referred to as the mesothelium

- **Endoderm origin** – develop into the inner linings of blood vessels, and referred to as the vascular endothelium

In general, the main function of epithelial tissue is to line, physically separate and compartmentalise various areas of the body from each other, and from the outside environment.

However, each type of epithelial tissue is also highly specialised to perform other functions too, depending on their location in the body.

Wherever their location in the body, and whatever their function, all epithelial tissues share the following features:

- All the cells are tightly joined together, so that the tissue forms a continuous sheet
- The tissue lies on a sub-layer of connective tissue fibres, which is called the **basement membrane** at the point where the two tissue types are in contact with each other
- The basement membrane allows attachment of the epithelial tissue to the underlying structures, it provides support and it also separates the epithelium from the underlying vascular connective tissue, called the **lamina propria**

The various types of epithelial tissue are classified according to the shape of the individual cells and whether the cells occur in one or more layers.

The shape classification is as follows:

- **Squamous** – appearing microscopically as flattened, plate-like cells
- **Cuboidal** – appearing cube-like, as the name suggests, with roughly equal width and height dimensions
- **Columnar** – appearing as tall, rectangular cells, where their height is greater than their width

The layer classification is as follows:

- **Simple epithelium** – a single layer of cells
- **Pseudostratified epithelium** – a single layer of cells that appears microscopically to be composed of several cell layers – this occurs due to variations in the size of the cells present, giving a falsely layered appearance
- **Stratified epithelium** – a truly layered tissue, consisting of two or more individual layers of cells

In addition, some epithelial tissues have a tough, waterproof covering of a protein called **keratin**, which makes the tissue impervious to bacterial invasion, and also better able to withstand frictional trauma. These tissues are referred to as **keratinised epithelia**.

Some examples of various epithelial tissues and their adaptations for specific functions are given in Table 1.1.

The general types of epithelial tissue are illustrated in Figure 1.4.

Table 1.1 Epithelial tissues and their functions.

Epithelial type	Functions	Examples
Simple squamous	Provide thin layer to allow the easy movement of molecules across them from one area to another	Alveoli of the lungs to allow gaseous exchange to occur Vascular endothelium to allow movement of chemicals into, and out of, the blood stream
Simple cuboidal	Provide a thin but more robust layer of single cells, often lining the ducts of glands and involved with secretion	Salivary glands Other exocrine glands
Simple cuboidal	Not lining a duct but allowing secretion directly into blood vessels	Islets of Langerhans in the pancreas Other endocrine glands
Simple columnar	Provide a thin but robust layer of cells, allowing both secretion and absorption	Small intestines Kidneys
Pseudostratified columnar	Some are further specialised by having the surface covered with microscopic hairs or cilia	Respiratory system, except the alveoli
Stratified squamous, keratinised and non-keratinised	Provide protection from chemical and physical trauma and from bacterial invasion	Parts of the oral cavity Surface of the skin

Connective tissue

This tissue develops both from the neuroectoderm and the mesoderm layers of the early embryo.

Like epithelial tissue, it has many specialised types as well as some basic common features across those types.

Examples of connective tissues are:

- Sub-layers of the skin and oral mucosa
- Cartilage
- Bone
- Blood and blood cells
- Lymph
- Dentine

The functions of connective tissue are many and varied.

In general, the tissue appears microscopically to be composed of cells spaced apart and suspended in a **matrix** of intercellular substance and fibres, with a vascular supply running through. The only exception is cartilage, which is not vascularised.

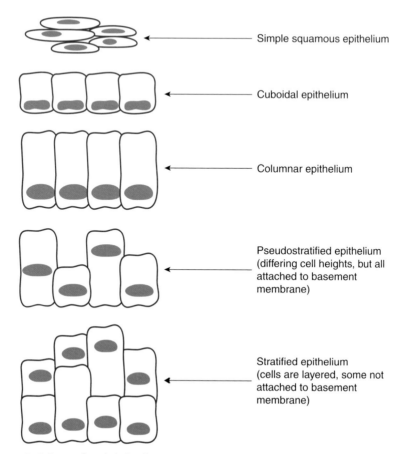

Figure 1.4 Types of epithelial cells.

The commonest cells found in all connective tissue are **fibroblasts,** which produce the intercellular substance and some of the fibres found in the matrix. Other cells which may be present will vary depending on the type of connective tissue concerned:

- Cartilage will contain **chondroblasts,** from which it is formed, and mature **chondrocytes**
- Similarly, bone will contain **osteoblasts** and **osteocytes**
- Blood, blood cells and lymph are discussed in detail in Chapter 2
- Dentine of teeth will contain **odontoblasts**

The fibres present are composed of protein, and can be formed into **collagen** or **elastin,** or both.

Collagen gives strength and resistance to tearing to the tissue, while elastin allows the tissue to stretch and reform without damage. Both are found in various areas of the oral cavity.

The connective tissues of greatest importance to the DCP are dentine and the periodontal ligament and are discussed in detail in Chapters 8 and 9, respectively.

ORGANS AND SYSTEMS

The organs and body systems relevant to the DCP are discussed in detail in Chapter 2 (CVS system), Chapter 3 (respiratory system), Chapter 4 (digestive system) and Chapter 5 (nervous system).

For the sake of completeness, the ten body systems present in humans are summarised in Table 1.2.

Table 1.2 The body systems.

System	Composed of	Functions
Cardiovascular	Heart, blood vessels, blood	Transport of blood to lungs for oxygenation Transport of oxygenated blood to body Transport of deoxygenated blood back to lungs
Respiratory	Nose, throat, larynx, trachea, lungs	Exchange of oxygen and carbon dioxide between the body and the atmosphere
Digestive	Mouth, salivary glands, pharynx, oesophagus, stomach, intestines, pancreas, liver, gall bladder	Digest, process and absorb nutrients from food Excrete waste products
Nervous	Brain, spinal cord, nerves, sensory organs	Gives consciousness Regulate and coordinate body activities
Musculoskeletal	Bone, cartilage, tendons, ligaments, joints, skeletal muscle	Support and protect internal organs Allows movement
Immune	White blood cells, lymph, spleen, bone marrow, thymus gland	Defend against infection Produces red and white blood cells
Endocrine	All glands that secrete hormones	Regulate and coordinate body workings
Urinary	Kidneys, ureter, bladder, urethra	Regulate blood plasma Excrete waste products
Reproductive	Male or female sex organs	Reproduction for the continuation of the species
Integumentary	Skin	Protect against injury and dehydration Maintain body temperature

The interaction of all the body systems to maintain life allows the continual production of energy by food digestion. This energy is used by the human body to carry out the following tasks for survival:

- Maintain body temperature above or below that of the surroundings; this is a particular ability of all mammals (including humans) and is referred to as **homeostasis**
- Produce movement to allow hunting for food (although for the majority of humans this is more likely to occur as a trip to the supermarket)
- The gathering and digestion of food will allow the production of more energy still
- Allows reproduction to occur for the survival of the species

DISEASE PROCESSES

Having given a basic overview of cell biology and tissue types, the DCP is now in a position to understand the generalities of disease and disease processes. This will give a better understanding of how illness and disease affect the body, as described in the following chapters.

In particular, an overview of the role of micro-organisms in disease processes is discussed.

Micro-organisms that have the capability of producing a disease are referred to as **pathogenic organisms,** or **pathogens,** as opposed to those that cannot cause illness or disease, which are called **non-pathogens.**

When pathogens attack the body, they may have several effects on the body cells and tissues, causing any of the following reactions:

- **Infection** – the actual invasion of the body cells by the pathogens, resulting in an **inflammatory response** of the cells, which produces the five signs of inflammation: **heat, swelling, pain, redness and loss of function**
- **Ulcer** – a shallow break in the skin or mucous membrane, leaving a raw and painful circular base that may bleed when touched
- **Cyst** – an abnormal sac of fluid that develops within the body tissues over a period of time
- **Tumour** – a swelling within any body tissue due to an uncontrolled and abnormal overgrowth of the body cells; when the swelling causes no harm other than displacing any surrounding structures it is called **benign,** but when the swelling invades and damages the surrounding structures it is called **malignant,** and is usually referred to as **cancer**

Response of the body to attack by pathogens

The body has three natural lines of defence against attack by pathogens, which in fit and healthy individuals are often enough to prevent the development of a serious illness:

- **Intact skin and mucous membrane,** which acts as a physical barrier against the pathogens, preventing them from entering the body
- **Surface secretions** that help to dilute and neutralise the pathogens and their poisons (**toxins**), such as:
  - Saliva in the mouth
  - Gastric juice in the stomach
  - Sweat on the skin
  - Tears in the eyes
- **Inflammatory response** if the body tissues are breached and they have to actively fight off the pathogens

The pathogens are more likely to be successful in developing into a disease process in individuals who are not fit and healthy when their body is attacked, as they may be unable to defend themselves, so that they become ill.

Those most likely to suffer are the following:

- **Elderly** – the functioning of the body cells in older patients is not as efficient as when they were younger as cells and tissues wear out with age and cannot be replaced as easily, and other age-related disorders may be present that affect the ability of the body to repair itself
- **Young children** – including babies, whose natural immune systems will not be functioning fully for some time, so they are more prone to developing diseases after attacks by pathogens, as well as not having received their full vaccination programme until older
- **Debilitated** – those patients of any age who are said to be **immuno-compromised** because they have an underlying illness that affects the ability of their immune system to fight off pathogens; this includes the following:
  - Diabetics
  - Those suffering from a range of illnesses such as leukaemia, kidney failure, AIDS and various cancers
  - Those taking drugs that act to suppress their immune systems due to organ transplant or cancer treatment

Inflammatory response

If the body tissues are breached by the pathogen, then an inflammatory response occurs.

This is the normal reaction of the body to exposure to an irritant such as an infective micro-organism, but it may also occur when exposed to physical and chemical irritants such as cuts, fire burns, chemical burns or poisons.

Microscopically, the reaction of the body is the same:

- Huge increase in the blood flow to the affected area, so that many leucocytes (white blood cells) can be transported there to fight the pathogens
- The sudden increase in blood volume in the area will cause the tissues to appear **red** and **swollen**, and feel **hot** to the touch
- The swollen tissues will also press against the surrounding nerve cells, causing **pain,** and the affected area will then become too painful to use, resulting in **loss of function**
- Leucocytes pass out of the capillaries and into the invaded body tissues to fight the pathogens by surrounding and eating them
- They are helped by the movement of blood plasma into the tissues, containing antibodies and antitoxins that act to neutralise the poisons produced by the pathogens
- Toxin production by the pathogens may be severe enough to cause a rise in body temperature from the normal 37°C, indicating an intense infection
- During the battle, both leucocytes and pathogens are killed, and their debris collects to form **pus** in the body tissues
- If the pus remains contained in the area of invasion it forms an **abscess,** but if it manages to spread into the surrounding tissues it is called **cellulitis**
- When the inflammatory process occurs as mentioned previously, it is described as **acute infection,** but when it occurs over a long period of time with few of the symptoms (especially pain) being evident, it is described as **chronic infection**
- If the infecting micro-organism is very powerful and difficult for the inflammatory response to control, it is described as **virulent**
- The elderly, the young and the debilitated may be unable to fight off an infection without the use of drugs such as **antibiotics, antivirals or antifungals,** and these may also have to be used in healthy individuals when a virulent organism is involved

When the inflammatory response occurs in the absence of micro-organisms (such as when exposed to physical or chemical irritants), no infection will occur, no pus will form and the body tissues will repair any damage caused by the irritant.

Tissue repair

Once the inflammatory response has overcome the infecting micro-organisms, or the physical or chemical irritant has been removed, the body will repair itself. New leucocytes will travel to the area and remove any damaged or dead tissue, and they will then lay down a temporary layer of repair cells called **granulation tissue.**

This consists of basic tissue cells and capillaries that form a fibrous framework for the more specialised tissue cells to grow and develop onto. So if the damage occurred in skin, skin cells will be formed; if in bone, bone cells will be formed, and so on.

If a chronic infection is persistently present, the body's attempts to repair the damage will only be partially successful, and a state will exist where tissue is being repaired at the same time as chronic infection is still present.

This is the usual case with infections such as **periodontal disease.**

The infecting micro-organisms are never completely eradicated, the chronic infection is always present and its severity swings between low grade and held at bay, with intermittent acute episodes that require treatment and drug therapy to overcome.

IMMUNITY

The immune system is composed of a complex network of various components throughout the body:

- **Bone marrow,** especially that in the pelvis and the sternum
- **Thymus gland,** in the upper chest area
- **Spleen,** in the upper abdomen
- **Lymph nodes,** throughout the body
- **Lymphoid tissues,** such as the tonsils and adenoids of the pharyngeal area
- **Some leucocytes,** particularly T lymphocytes and B lymphocytes

During the inflammatory response, certain leucocytes are not involved in fighting the micro-organisms, but are stimulated to release **antibodies and antitoxins** into the blood plasma instead.

The stimulation occurs because these leucocytes recognise the invaders as being foreign to the normal body tissues; they are identified as **antigens.**

Other antigens that will cause a similar response are:

- Transplanted organs
- Foreign bodies
- Toxins from plant and animal tissues
- Incompatible blood transfusions

The antibodies and antitoxins are quite specific for an invading micro-organism, and some are present from birth by being inherited randomly; this is called **natural immunity.**

Others are present at birth in the newborn due to the specific inheritance of a mother's own antibodies and antitoxins; this is called **passive immunity.**

Once a micro-organism has been encountered and the infection fought off, the necessary antibodies and antitoxins will remain in the individual's blood for life to prevent any recurrence of the same infection. This is called **acquired immunity**.

Unfortunately, this does not occur for every micro-organism and in addition, many of them (especially viruses) can go through a process called **mutation**, where they change their chemical make-up slightly and effectively produce a new variation of a disease.

The individual will then have to be exposed to this new variant before suitable antibodies and antitoxins can be made by their leucocytes. Until then, they are at risk of being infected by the new variant pathogen.

Viruses that mutate relatively easily and develop new strains on a regular basis include those responsible for **influenza**.

Where acquired immunity is possible for a micro-organism, it can be produced artificially by injecting the individual with a dose of the dead micro-organisms; this will stimulate the leucocytes to develop the necessary antibodies and antitoxins to fight off the disease, but without actually infecting the individual with that disease. This is called **vaccination**.

In this way, individuals can be protected against serious and fatal infections without having to be exposed to, and survive, the actual attack.

By the close-up and hands-on nature of dental treatment, all members of the dental team are exposed to many infections daily and are at risk of catching any of them.

Consequently, all clinical dental personnel must be vaccinated against the following:

- **Hepatitis B**
- **MMR** – measles, mumps and rubella (German measles)
- **Tuberculosis** and **whooping cough** (pertussis)
- **Poliomyelitis**
- **Tetanus** and **diphtheria**
- **Chickenpox** (if not already naturally immune)
- **Meningitis**

Some serious and fatal diseases have no vaccination available at present, and one of the most important ones in relation to the dental team is AIDS.

This is because it is transmitted mainly by blood, and many dental procedures produce bleeding.

Avoidance of infection by any micro-organism can only occur if procedures are in place within the dental workplace with regard to the following:

- Staff vaccination
- Use of protective wear during treatment and cleaning procedures
- Use of single-use disposables where possible
- Correct cleaning methods

Allergy

Occasionally, the immune system overreacts in its response to the presence of an antigen, with sudden swelling of the tissues and copious production of fluids occurring.

This is called hypersensitivity and produces an allergic reaction.

It can range in severity from a mild rash to a full anaphylactic shock episode, which is potentially fatal.

Often, individuals prone to an allergic reaction will already suffer from disorders such as asthma, eczema or hay fever, so they are able to be identified from their medical history.

During dental treatment, areas of caution in an effort to avoid a hypersensitivity reaction involve the non-use of **latex products** (such as gloves and rubber dam sheets), and the non-prescribing of some drugs, especially the antibiotic **penicillin** and its derivatives.

ANATOMICAL NOMENCLATURE

As a final introduction and overview to the areas of anatomy and physiology, the DCP needs to be familiar with and understand the specific terminology used when describing anatomical features.

It is a system similar to that used when charting the dentition, which is an area of great familiarity to all DCPs, where each tooth surface has a specific name to identify it in relation to the midline of each dental arch (see Chapter 8).

Anatomical nomenclature appears slightly more complicated than this, as it is used in reference to the body in three dimensions, with the key points for the DCP as follows:

- **Median plane** – an imaginary line through the exact centre of the whole body, dividing it into left and right sides
- **Frontal plane** – an imaginary line at right angles to the median plane, dividing the whole body into front and back sides
- **Horizontal plane** – an imaginary line at right angles to both the median and frontal planes (so horizontal to the ground), lying at any height of the body and dividing it into upper and lower sections
- **Surface depth** – an additional descriptive term used to indicate the depth of a structure in relation to the surface of the body

The planes described are illustrated in Figure 1.5.

When describing anatomical structures in relation to the median plane, those closest to the centre line are **medial** while those furthest away are **lateral**. Relevant examples are the **medial and lateral pterygoid muscles** of mastication (see Chapter 7).

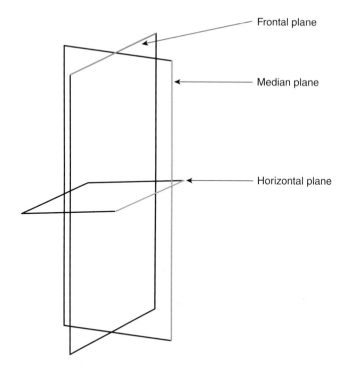

Frontal plane

Median plane

Horizontal plane

Figure 1.5 Anatomical planes.

When describing anatomical structures in relation to the frontal plane, those in front of the plane are **anterior** while those behind the plane are **posterior**. Relevant examples are the **anterior and posterior digastric muscles**, members of the suprahyoid group of muscles.

When describing anatomical structures in relation to a horizontal plane, those above the plane are **superior** while those below the plane are **inferior**. Relevant examples are the **superior and inferior dental nerves** supplying the teeth and their surrounding structures.

So, when combining the nomenclature together, the position of any anatomical structure can be exactly described in relation to its surrounding structures, in terminology that is understandable in any language.

The names of muscles, bones and nerves may initially appear complicated and onerous to those studying anatomy, but when the nomenclature is fully understood, those names describe the exact anatomical location of the structure in the minimum number of words.

Relevant examples are the following:

- **Anterior superior dental nerve** – supplying the front, upper teeth and surrounding structures
- **Posterior superior dental nerve** – supplying the back, upper teeth and surrounding structures
- **Inferior dental nerve** – supplying the lower teeth and surrounding structures

Finally, when describing anatomical structures in relation to their surface depth, those closest to the surface are said to be **superficial** while those furthest from the surface are said to be **deep**.

Relevant examples are the **superficial and deep lobes of the submandibular salivary gland**. The former lies outside the surrounding muscles and is palpable externally, while the latter lies beneath the muscles (see Chapter 10).

Chapter 2

Cardiovascular system

The cardiovascular system is composed of the following:
- The **heart**
- Blood vessels carrying blood away from the heart – **arteries and arterioles**
- Blood vessels carrying blood to the heart – **veins and venules**
- Microscopic blood vessels connecting these two systems together – **capillaries**
- Blood – consisting of various cells suspended in a fluid – **plasma**

The whole system is sealed and enclosed, and runs in a similar fashion to a central heating system in a house.

In this analogy, the radiators in each room represent the organs of the body, the pipes to and from the radiators represent the blood vessels, the boiler represents the lungs and the water pump represents the heart.

When the pump is switched on it moves cold water to the boiler to be heated, and the hot water is then pumped through the pipes to all the radiators to heat the house. As the water in the radiators loses the heat, it is pumped back to the boiler to be re-heated again.

The circulation of the blood throughout the body is represented diagrammatically in Figure 2.1.

THE HEART – GROSS ANATOMY

The heart is a muscular pumping organ situated in the chest cavity, or **thorax**.

In gross anatomy, it is composed of four chambers – two on the left and two on the right, with no natural communication between the two sides except in the foetus. The ventricles are separated by the **interventricular septum**.

The **left** side is concerned with **oxygenated blood only**, and the **right** side with **deoxygenated blood only**.

The two upper chambers are called the **atria** and the two lower chambers are called the **ventricles**. The atria receive blood from the body through various

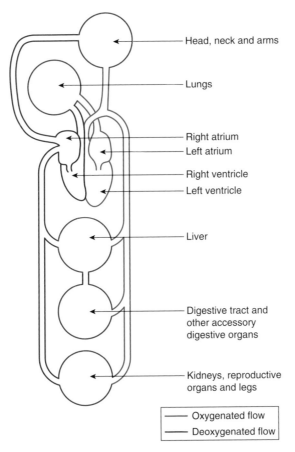

Head, neck and arms

Lungs

Right atrium
Left atrium

Right ventricle
Left ventricle

Liver

Digestive tract and
other accessory
digestive organs

Kidneys, reproductive
organs and legs

——— Oxygenated flow
——— Deoxygenated flow

Figure 2.1 Body circulation.

veins, while the ventricles deliver blood from within the heart to the body through various arteries.

In effect, the cardiovascular system operates as two interlinked circulatory systems; one taking blood to and from the lungs only – **the pulmonary circulation,** and the other taking blood to and from the rest of the body – **the systemic system.**

The gross anatomy of the heart and the passage of blood within it are illustrated in Figure 2.2.

Following the blood flow from the body, through the heart to the lungs and back, and then out to the body again, the sequence is as follows:

- Deoxygenated blood from the body travels to the **right atrium** in the large veins called the **inferior and superior venae cavae**
- It is pumped from the right atrium to the **right ventricle** within the heart through the one-way **tricuspid valve,** which prevents back flow

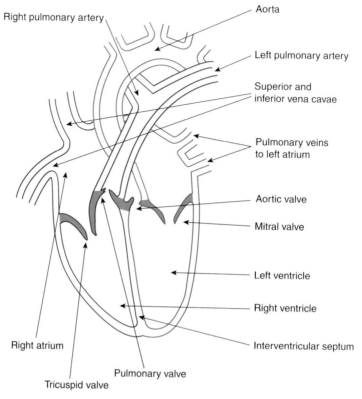

Figure 2.2 Gross anatomy of the heart.

- Then from the right ventricle to the lungs in the **pulmonary artery** – the only artery to carry deoxygenated blood
- The **pulmonary valve** prevents back flow of blood back into the right ventricle
- The blood is oxygenated in the lungs
- Oxygenated blood travels from the lungs to the **left atrium** through the **pulmonary veins** – the only veins to carry oxygenated blood
- It is pumped from the left atrium to the **left ventricle** within the heart, passing through the one-way **mitral valve** to prevent back flow
- Finally, it is pumped from the left ventricle out of the heart to the rest of body via the **aorta**
- This is the largest of the arteries in the body, and back flow is prevented by the **aortic valve**
- As the aorta leaves the heart, it immediately branches as the **coronary arteries**, which supply the heart muscle itself with oxygenated blood
- Some of the next branches are the **carotid arteries**, which supply the head and neck region

THE HEART – MICROSCOPIC ANATOMY

The muscle tissue present in the heart (**cardiac muscle**) is unique and quite different from that involved in body movement (skeletal muscle) or that around hollow cavities within the body (smooth muscle).

Cardiac muscle has the ability to continue to contract and relax rhythmically, even when it is separated from its nerve supply and is, therefore, not being acted upon by electrical impulses from nerve tissue. In addition, it also does not become tired after a time and cease to contract, like other muscles do. No other muscle tissue has these abilities.

Collectively, the heart wall muscle is known as the **myocardium,** while the inner surface of the heart is lined by a thin layer of epithelial tissue called the **endocardium.**

The endocardium is an unbroken layer of tissue that runs into the inner surface lining of the blood vessels, called the **vascular endothelium.**

THE CARDIAC CYCLE

The heartbeat, or cardiac cycle, occurs about seventy times per minute in the average resting adult human.

It begins in a specialised group of muscle cells on the outer wall of the right atrium, called the **sino-atrial node,** or 'pacemaker'.

These specialised cells receive electrical stimulation from two sets of nerves in the brain, one set speeds up the heart rate and the other set slows it down – so the rate of the heart beat is regulated to allow both exercise and rest, as necessary.

The full cycle occurs as follows:

- Once stimulated at the pacemaker, waves of electrical activity spread quickly across both atria, causing them to **contract** – this is called **atrial systole**
- This pumps their blood contents into the ventricles, where it is prevented from back flowing by the tricuspid and mitral valves
- The initial electrical wave stops at this point, after stimulating a second node on the bottom edge of the right atrium, called the **atrio-ventricular node**
- Electrical impulses from the second node travel in a bundle of specialised cells (**bundle of His**) lying in the interventricular septum, down to the apex of the heart **without** spreading across the surfaces of the ventricles
- Once at the apex, the electrical impulse is transmitted from the bottom of the ventricles upwards in specialised fibres (**Purkinje fibres**), causing ventricular contraction in this same direction – this is called **ventricular systole**

CARDIOVASCULAR SYSTEM

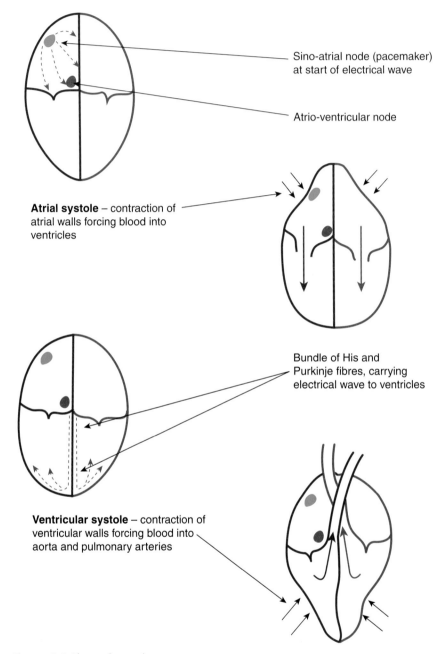

Sino-atrial node (pacemaker)
at start of electrical wave

Atrio-ventricular node

Atrial systole – contraction of
atrial walls forcing blood into
ventricles

Bundle of His and
Purkinje fibres, carrying
electrical wave to ventricles

Ventricular systole – contraction of
ventricular walls forcing blood into
aorta and pulmonary arteries

Figure 2.3 The cardiac cycle.

- The directional nature of the ventricular contraction enables their blood contents to be pumped upwards and out of the heart into the aorta and pulmonary arteries
- Back flow is prevented by the aortic and pulmonary valves

The various valves within the heart are non-muscular structures; they open and close purely due to the fluid pressure differences produced during the contractions of the various heart chambers.

The rhythmic opening and closing of the valves are the heart beat sounds made audible by the use of a stethoscope during clinical examination.

These are often described as 'lub dup' – 'lub' when the tricuspid and mitral valves simultaneously close, and 'dup' when the aortic and pulmonary valves simultaneously close.

The cardiac cycle is shown in Figure 2.3.

BLOOD VESSELS – FUNCTIONS

The three broad types of blood vessel – arteries, veins and capillaries – have each developed to best carry out their particular functions.

Arteries and arterioles (small arteries) specifically transport oxygenated blood from the heart to the body (except the pulmonary artery) and nutrients from the digestive system to the body tissues.

Oxygen is required by all of the body cells to produce energy to work, and nutrients are required for growth and repair.

Veins and venules (small veins) specifically transport deoxygenated blood from the body to the lungs via the heart (except the pulmonary vein) and collect waste products from body tissues to be excreted by the urinary system.

The gaseous waste product of respiration (breathing) is carbon dioxide, while many waste products are produced when nutrients are used by cells and tissues for growth and repair. All these waste products must be eliminated by the body to avoid the development of toxic and acidic conditions, which are damaging to healthy tissues.

Capillaries are the microscopic vessels where these various gaseous and nutrient exchanges occur, lying as networks of vessels that interconnect the arterial and venous sides of the circulatory system.

BLOOD VESSELS – MICROSCOPIC ANATOMY

Arteries and arterioles

These vessels are made up of three layers of tissue, as follows:

- **Endothelium** – the inner layer of the vessel and in direct contact with the blood

- **Smooth muscle** – the middle layer of the vessel and surrounds the whole of it with a circular muscle layer, giving the blood vessel strength and the ability to avoid collapse. In the smaller arterioles, more smooth muscle than elastic tissue is present to allow these smaller vessels to regulate the blood flow in their area of supply
- **Elastic layer** – the outer layer of the vessel and gives it the ability to stretch as a pulse of blood surges through, and then tighten again to ensure the blood flows onwards between heart beats

Those arteries closest to the heart tend to have a thicker elastic layer than the smaller arterioles, so that they are better able to withstand the force of the blood surge as it first leaves the heart, without rupturing.

At the point between the end of ventricular systole and the beginning of the next atrial systole, the blood surge is continued along the length of the arteries to the body tissues by the sequential tightening action of the elastic layer.

The point between the two systoles, when the ventricles are relaxed, is called **diastole**.

So, the maximum pressure of the blood in the arteries occurs during the peak of ventricular contraction, or systole, while the minimum pressure occurs at the end of ventricular contraction, or diastole.

Hence, blood pressure is recorded as systolic pressure over diastolic pressure, and in a healthy adult at rest it is usually around 120/80.

It is measured as millimetres of mercury, with a sphygmomanometer and a stethoscope.

Capillaries

The arterial blood vessels become smaller and smaller, the further they are from the heart, being called arterioles when they are less than a certain diameter. As they arrive at the tissues they are supplying, they become smaller still and branch repeatedly, until they give rise to capillaries.

Capillaries have the following features:

- **Endothelium** – made up of just a single layer of cells, so that gases, nutrients and waste products can pass across them easily in an exchange mechanism
- **No muscle layer** – this would prevent the exchange mechanism from occurring
- **No elastic layer** – this is not required as the blood flow in these vessels is no longer pulsatile, and again, it would prevent the exchange mechanism from occurring

It is in the capillary beds that the oxygen inspired in the lungs passes out of the circulatory system and into the body tissues to be used to create energy by the cells.

At the same time, carbon dioxide passes from the body tissues into the capillaries to be transported back to the lungs and exhaled. It is formed as the waste product of the cell activities during energy production.

This transfer of the two gases within the capillary beds is called **internal respiration.**

Nutrients and waste materials are exchanged in a similar manner, by passing out of the capillaries and forming **tissue fluid,** before being selectively absorbed by the body tissues. Any fluid then not reabsorbed by the capillaries enters a different set of vessels, called the **lymph vessels.**

The lymph system acts as a safety mechanism, by draining all unwanted materials from the body tissues rather than allowing them to accumulate there, thereby reducing the efficiency of the normal exchange mechanism.

The lymph fluid so formed is transported through various **lymph nodes throughout the body,** before being returned to the circulatory system via the large veins draining the head and neck region.

While passing through the lymph nodes, any small particles, including micro-organisms, are destroyed by defence cells. Similarly, toxins from waste products are neutralised, and lymph nodes are also involved in antibody production.

The relationship between the capillary beds and the lymph system is shown in Figure 2.4.

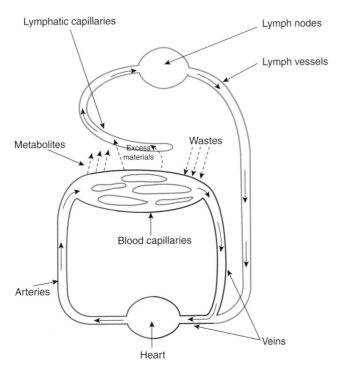

Figure 2.4 Relationship of the capillary beds and the lymph system.

Veins and venules

These vessels are similar in structure to arteries, being composed of the same three tissue layers, but they are much thinner overall and are therefore able to distend (enlarge).

The larger veins of the limbs also possess valves at regular intervals along their length. These allow blood to flow unimpeded towards the heart, while preventing back flow in the opposite direction.

The structure of each of the blood vessels is illustrated in Figure 2.5.

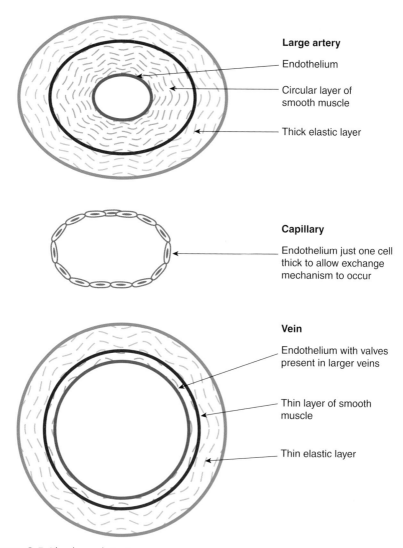

Large artery

Endothelium

Circular layer of smooth muscle

Thick elastic layer

Capillary

Endothelium just one cell thick to allow exchange mechanism to occur

Vein

Endothelium with valves present in larger veins

Thin layer of smooth muscle

Thin elastic layer

Figure 2.5 Blood vessel structure.

BLOOD – COMPOSITION AND FUNCTIONS

Although considered by some to be a specialised type of connective tissue, blood is unique in that it exists as cells within a fluid.

The fluid component of blood is called **plasma**, a clear pale yellow fluid composed mainly of water (95%), and with various proteins, mineral ions and organic molecules such as sugars making up the rest.

Suspended in the plasma are various blood cells, which are transported around the body within the circulatory system:

- **Erythrocytes** – red blood cells, which give blood its red colour
- **Leucocytes** – white blood cells, which consist of three major categories of cell
- **Thrombocytes** – platelets, which are actually fragmented portions of other larger cells originating in the bone marrow

All of the different types of blood cell are formed from a group of specialised **stem cells** within the bone marrow. Stem cells have the ability to develop and differentiate into any of the different types of blood cell at any one time, depending on the needs of the body and/or the presence of any disorders affecting the body.

The particular bone marrow sites of stem cell production in adults are the pelvis, the spinal vertebrae, the collar bones and shoulder bones (clavicles and scapulae), the skull and the ends of the long limb bones.

Details of the various blood cells are shown in Table 2.1.

Table 2.1 Blood cells.

Cell type	Production site	Functions
Erythrocytes	Bone marrow	Transport of oxygen from the lungs to the body tissues Transport of carbon dioxide from the body tissues to the lungs
Leucocytes		
Granulocytes	Bone marrow	Segregation of bacteria and other foreign particles from body tissues Production of histamine Antihistamine properties in areas of inflammation
Monocytes	Bone marrow	Destruction of bacteria and other segregated particles
Lymphocytes	Bone marrow Lymph tissue Spleen	Production of antibodies
Platelets	Bone marrow	Initiate blood clotting at injury sites

Together, the various blood cells have a variety of functions as follows, with their ability to carry out these functions being enabled by the transport system of the blood plasma:

- Carriage of oxygen from the lungs to the body tissues
- Carriage of carbon dioxide from the body tissues to the lungs
- Absorption of nutrients from the digestive system and transport to the body tissues
- Transport of waste products to the liver and urinary system
- Transport of hormones to various sites throughout the body
- Defence against diseases

The microscopic appearance of the various blood cells is shown in Figure 2.6.

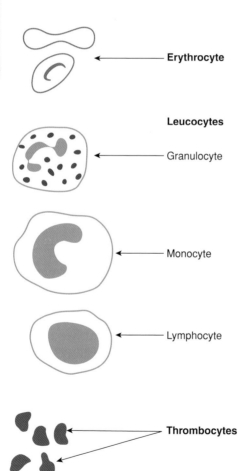

Erythrocyte

Leucocytes

Granulocyte

Monocyte

Lymphocyte

Thrombocytes

Figure 2.6 Types of blood cell.

Erythrocytes – specific structure and roles

Erythrocytes form the majority of the cells present in blood, and appear microscopically as anucleate, biconcave discs – effectively 'doughnut shaped' and without a nucleus.

The main constituent of the erythrocyte is the protein **haemoglobin**, and this binds very strongly to oxygen and enables the cells to carry out their main function – the transport of oxygen around the body.

Chemically, each haemoglobin molecule can bind to four oxygen molecules to form **oxyhaemoglobin,** but at any one time there will also be a small number of oxygen molecules dissolved in the blood plasma.

Erythrocytes 'pick up' oxygen molecules as they pass through the capillaries within the lungs, where the oxygen concentration is high, and then release them in areas of low oxygen concentration within the tissue capillaries, during the process of internal respiration.

The loss of the oxygen molecules converts the oxyhaemoglobin to a new compound called **deoxyhaemoglobin.**

Visibly, oxyhaemoglobin gives arterial blood its bright red colour, while deoxyhaemoglobin gives venous blood its deep purple colour.

The erythrocyte cells are formed within the bone marrow and have around a 4-month lifespan, after which they are removed from the circulation as they pass through the liver and spleen. Their haemoglobin content is efficiently recycled, and forms part of the structure of new erythrocytes as they are formed in the bone marrow.

The erythrocytes are constantly being produced and replaced in this way, and the process can be controlled so that production is accelerated as required by the body.

This happens especially so following blood loss from haemorrhage, or blood donation.

In contrast to oxygen, the majority of the carbon dioxide formed as a waste product during cell metabolism is not carried within the erythrocytes, but travels as a chemical ion called **bicarbonate** within the blood plasma.

The amount of carbon dioxide transported in this form to the lungs for removal depends on the amount of oxyhaemoglobin present in the surrounding circulation.

Where oxyhaemoglobin levels are low, the blood is able to carry more carbon dioxide – so in the body tissues where cells are metabolising and producing much carbon dioxide, large amounts of the gas are converted to bicarbonate ions and carried away from the area in the blood plasma.

When this blood plasma reaches the capillaries within the lungs, the high levels of oxyhaemoglobin here cause the system to 'offload' the carbon dioxide, and it is removed from the lungs during expiration (breathing out).

Leucocytes – specific structure and roles

Leucocytes occur in far fewer numbers in blood than erythrocytes, and they occur in three main categories:

- **Granulocytes**
- **Monocytes**
- **Lymphocytes**

All three categories of cell contain a nucleus, the shape of which is used microscopically to identify each particular white cell, and all are involved with the defence of the body against disease.

Granulocytes form the greatest number of leucocytes in the blood at any one time. They exist in a variety of cell types but all are formed from stem cells within the bone marrow. Some are able to leave the blood stream by squeezing between the endothelial cells of venules, and attack bacteria directly within the tissue cells themselves.

Their collective roles as part of the body's immune system are as follows:

- Engulfing and digestion of bacteria (**phagocytosis**)
- **Antihistamine effect** during allergic responses and at sites of inflammation
- Production of **histamine**, causing localised effect of vasodilatation (increased local blood flow)

Monocytes are the largest in size of the leucocytes, and although they are formed in the bone marrow they spend their life in other tissues of the body, such as the brain, liver and spleen.

They mature in these tissues to become large phagocytes, or **macrophages**, and are able to engulf and destroy bacteria and other foreign bodies that could harm the body tissues.

Lymphocytes occur as one of two types:

- **B lymphocytes** – formed and mature in the bone marrow, and produce specific antibodies
- **T lymphocytes** – formed in the bone marrow, mature in the thymus gland, lymph tissue and the spleen, and are involved in immune response mechanisms

The T lymphocytes are particularly important in recognising body cells that have been infected by a virus, and destroying those cells and therefore the virus within.

All viruses require a **host cell** to invade and replicate in, they cannot replicate and cause their specific viral infection otherwise. Any body cell can be invaded and act as the host cell, providing a safe environment for the virus to replicate itself and invade surrounding cells and tissues, causing a viral infection.

Once recognised and targeted by T lymphocytes though, the infected host cell is stimulated to destroy itself by being exposed to poisons (toxins) released by the lymphocyte. This process prevents the virus from becoming established, and causing an overwhelming viral infection.

Thrombocytes – specific structure and roles

Platelets, or thrombocytes, are actually fragments of larger cells found in the bone marrow called **megakaryocytes**, which, like the other blood cells, are formed from stem cells. The platelets have no particular shape, they usually have no nucleus and they survive within the circulatory system for approximately just 10 days.

The role of thrombocytes is to physically plug a tear in a blood vessel wall, so that blood loss through an injury is reduced while the blood clotting mechanism is activated, and the blood is able to coagulate.

The process of preventing blood loss from a damaged vessel, while enabling coagulation to occur at the injury site only, is called **haemostasis**.

Any injury causing damage to the endothelial lining of the blood vessel results in contraction of the muscle layer of the blood vessel itself, so that the damaged portion is 'squeezed shut' and blood flow is restricted in that area.

This is called **vasoconstriction**, and it can also be deliberately brought about by various chemicals, such as adrenaline and oxytocin. These agents are added to some local anaesthetic solutions used in dentistry, and the localised vasoconstriction they produce allows for a longer period of anaesthesia and reduced bleeding.

In addition to vasoconstriction, the damaged blood vessel also releases potent chemicals that become 'activated' (switched on) to begin the process of blood coagulation. Meantime, the exposed connective tissue of the blood vessel, lying beneath the endothelium, becomes sticky and allows platelets to adhere to it to form a **platelet plug**.

The resultant reduction in blood loss brought about by vasoconstriction and the formation of the platelet plug are only interim measures in the body's attempts not to bleed to death.

The most important event in avoiding catastrophic blood loss is for the body to form a stable blood clot by **coagulation**, to physically seal the injury site. The formation of the blood clot occurs via a complicated **coagulation pathway**, the details of which are beyond the remit of this text.

In simple terms, the pathway involves the sequential activation of various plasma proteins and other molecules (called **clotting factors**), in a similar manner to the 'knock-on' effect of a line of dominoes falling over. The end result is the conversion of the soluble plasma protein **fibrinogen** into the insoluble protein **fibrin**, by the action of the enzyme **thrombin**.

Fibrin is microscopically thread-like in appearance, and acts as a biological mesh at the injury site by physically trapping blood cells and plasma in the threads to form a blood clot. Once bleeding has ceased, the blood clot retracts and allows the damaged blood vessel to repair itself, and then ultimately the clot is broken down and removed from the area.

CVS MEDICAL CONDITIONS

Heart failure

This occurs when the pumping efficiency of the heart itself is inadequate, resulting in its inability to pump enough blood with each beat to allow the body to function normally, and to carry out its normal metabolic activities. It may involve either one of the ventricles, or both together.

Heart failure occurs either due to a problem with the heart itself, or due to a medical condition that increases the workload of the heart as it pumps blood around the body.

Those due to the heart itself are:

- **Myocardial infarction** – a 'heart attack', where there is a sudden reduction in the oxygenated blood supply to the heart itself through a coronary artery, often due to blockage by a blood clot (**thrombus**), and causing a section of the heart muscle itself to die – this is **acute heart failure**
- **Myocarditis** – inflammation of the heart muscle itself, usually as a result of a viral infection
- **Valvular disease** – affecting any of the heart valves so that the filling or emptying of the heart itself is inadequate, and it has to work harder to overcome the resistance to efficient blood movement that the diseased valve causes

Those due to a medical condition causing an increased heart workload are:

- **Angina** – a condition of **myocardial ischaemia** caused by the narrowing and partial blockage of the coronary arteries, due to the presence of fatty deposits or **atheromatous plaques**. When the heart workload increases, especially during exercise, the narrowed arteries are unable to supply sufficient oxygenated blood to the cardiac muscle, and symptoms similar to a heart attack are felt
- **Renal failure** – kidney failure results in an increased blood volume throughout the body due to excessive fluid retention as the kidneys fail to remove adequate water and sodium from the body by urinary excretion. The increased blood volume requires more work by the heart to pump it around the body, to the point where the coronary arteries are unable to supply sufficient oxygenated blood to the cardiac muscle, resulting in **myocardial ischaemia**
- **Hypertension** – raised blood pressure at rest (rather than during exercise) means that the heart has to pump more strongly to move blood from the left

ventricle into the aorta and so out to the body tissues, putting a constant strain on the cardiac muscle itself. In some cases, the coronary arteries are unable to supply sufficient oxygenated blood, and **myocardial ischaemia** develops

Oedema in heart failure

All the medical conditions described, except myocardial infarction, produce the condition of **chronic heart failure.**

This is characterised by varying degrees of breathlessness, tiredness and chest pain on exercise, rather than the sudden, crushing symptoms felt during a heart attack.

The myocardial ischaemia that occurs in chronic heart failure causes oxygenated blood flow to be diverted to the heart, the brain and the skeletal musculature, and away from other organs. Crucially, the reduced blood flow to the kidneys results in fluid retention, and this excess fluid tends to accumulate in the body tissues and is called **oedema.**

When the right side of the heart is failing (**right-sided heart failure**), the excess fluid will pool in the body peripheries, especially the ankles, and is referred to as **peripheral oedema.**

A more serious situation occurs when the left side of the heart is failing (**left-sided heart failure**), as the fluid accumulation occurs in the lungs themselves. The resulting **pulmonary oedema** reduces the effectiveness of the gas exchange mechanism within the lungs, reducing the availability of oxygen to the heart and other organs still further, and eventually death will occur.

Hypertension

Otherwise known as 'high blood pressure', hypertension is a commonly occurring cardiovascular condition that accounts for many deaths each year, usually due to complications affecting the various blood vessels of the body.

It is present when the blood pressure is recorded as persistently higher than usual, the accepted level being above 140/90. However, other factors are able to cause a raised systolic pressure above 140, including increasing age as well as anxiety, so a raised diastolic pressure above 90 is more relevant in the diagnosis of hypertension.

The two types of hypertension are:

- **Primary hypertension** – which occurs in the absence of other diseases or medical conditions, and is also referred to as **essential hypertension**
- **Secondary hypertension** – which occurs due to other diseases or medical conditions

The overall effect of hypertension is to force the heart to work harder to pump blood around the body, and to thicken the muscle layer of the blood vessel walls, causing their narrowing.

Primary hypertension accounts for the majority of cases, and is linked to various risk factors:

- Obesity
- Smoking and/or excessive alcohol intake
- Family history of cardiovascular conditions
- Increasing age
- Stress

Where possible, life-style changes play a key role in the treatment of hypertension, with or without the aid of medication.

Secondary hypertension is usually caused by any condition or disease that reduces blood flow to the kidneys, as they are then unable to regulate the volume of fluid within the body. If excess fluid is not excreted by the urinary system, the increased volume causes a pressure build-up throughout the body, and is recorded as a raised blood pressure.

Other causes of secondary hypertension include pregnancy and some vascular disorders, where the blood vessels themselves become narrowed and restrictive to normal blood flow, causing back pressure.

BLOOD CELL DISORDERS

Disorders of the various blood cell types will result in a reduction in their particular functions:

- **Erythrocyte disorders** – result in a reduction in the carriage and exchange of oxygen and carbon dioxide
- **Leucocyte disorders** – result in a reduction in the body's immune response mechanisms
- **Thrombocyte disorders** – result in a reduction in the ability of the blood to clot

Particular disorders that can occur for each of the blood cell types are as follows:

- **Erythrocytes**
  - **Anaemias** – caused by a reduced number of erythrocytes, resulting in a reduced oxygen carrying capacity of the blood
  - **Polycythaemia** – caused by overproduction of red blood cells, resulting in an increased viscosity (thick blood) and strain on the heart and kidneys, and an increased risk of stroke and deep vein thrombosis
- **Leucocytes**
  - **Leukaemias** – caused by large numbers of abnormal leucocytes in the blood, which are unable to function to protect the body from disease
  - **Leucopenia** – caused by a reduction in the numbers of white blood cells, leaving the body prone to infection

- Thrombocytes
  - **Thrombocytopenia** – caused by an overall reduction in the number of circulating platelets, eventually resulting in large blood loss after an injury, or even spontaneous blood loss

Thrombosis

A **thrombus**, or blood clot, can form within an intact blood vessel, as an abnormal occurrence.

This may happen when the blood flow in the vessel is slow and sluggish (such as in bed-bound patients), or in the presence of fatty deposits (**atheroma**) stuck to the inside of arterial walls, as occurs in **atherosclerosis.**

A thrombus that develops within an artery will reduce the oxygenated blood flow to the organ that it supplies; in severe cases, it may even block the blood flow completely.

In key arteries this can have serious consequences:

- **Coronary artery thrombosis** – supplying part of the heart and resulting in a **myocardial infarction**
- **Cerebral thrombosis** – supplying part of the brain and resulting in a **stroke**
- **Other key areas** – the loss of oxygenated blood supply to any organ or area of the body can potentially result in death of the tissue and the onset of gangrene
- **Thromboembolism** – when a fraction of the original thrombus breaks away and circulates in the blood stream to other key organs, most noticeably the lungs and causing a **pulmonary embolism**

A thrombus may also develop in a vein, especially the deep veins of the legs after a period of incapacity, such as following surgery, when the patient is bed-bound.

This is a **deep vein thrombosis** and is particularly serious, as displaced emboli from the original thrombus will travel in the venous circulation to the heart and then onto the lungs – causing a **pulmonary embolism.**

This reduces or even stops the blood flow to the affected lung, and can be fatal if not treated immediately.

CVS MEDICATIONS

Acute heart failure

The aims of drug therapy at the time of the 'heart attack' episode are to limit the size of damaged heart tissue that results, to prevent further clot formation and to limit the effects of the reduced oxygen supply:

- **Aspirin** – to prevent further clot formation by preventing platelet aggregation
- **Oxygen** – to increase oxygenation of the tissues

- **Clot busters** – various drugs to break down other circulating clots before they do further damage
- **Anticoagulants** – to prevent further thrombus formation, especially a deep vein thrombosis

Chronic heart failure

The aim of drug therapy is to reduce the workload of the heart:

- **Diuretics** – such as 'bendroflumethiazide', which reduce the volume of fluid that the heart is having to pump around the body by enabling the kidneys to function more efficiently and excrete it
- **Digoxin** – which improves the pumping efficiency of the heart

Angina

The aim of drug therapy to avoid an 'angina attack' is to reduce the work of the heart so that the reduced blood supply is able to meet the oxygen demands at the time:

- **Glyceryl trinitrate (GTN)** – opens the peripheral veins so that blood can pool here rather than all being pumped around the circulation, this then reduces the volume of blood returning to the heart and reduces its work load
- **Calcium antagonists** – act to relax the muscle layer of arteries so that they can dilate and allow more blood flow (include 'amilodipine', 'nifedipine' and 'verapamil')
- **Aspirin** – to reduce platelet aggregation in areas of atherosclerosis within the blood vessels, and so prevent thrombus formation

Sufferers on long-term aspirin therapy will have 'thin blood' and may bleed profusely after dental extractions. This can be avoided by temporarily stopping the medication prior to the extraction and by careful post-operative management of haemostasis using sutures and haemostatic sponges.

Some calcium antagonists, such as nifedipine, have several side effects, including the onset of gingival hyperplasia.

Patients may have to undergo repeated gingivectomy procedures when gingival overgrowth prevents adequate routine oral hygiene levels from being maintained.

The gingival hyperplasia is exacerbated, but not caused by, the presence of dental plaque.

Hypertension

The aim of drug therapy is to maintain a reduced blood pressure as a preventive measure, so that organ damage due to untreated hypertension is kept to a minimum:

- **Diuretics** – such as 'bendroflumethiazide', which reduce the volume of fluid that the heart is having to pump around the body, by enabling the kidneys to function more efficiently and excrete it
- **Calcium antagonists** – such as 'amlodipine', which act to relax the muscle layer of arteries to allow their dilation and allow more peripheral blood flow, so taking the strain off the heart
- **Propanolol and atenolol** – which slow the heart rate and the force of contraction, thereby reducing the cardiac output and lessening the strain on the heart

CARDIOVASCULAR SYSTEM

Chapter 3

Respiratory system

The respiratory system is composed of the following:

- The **lungs**
- Upper respiratory vessels that allow entry of atmospheric air into the respiratory system – **nose** (and mouth), **larynx** (and pharynx) and **trachea** (the windpipe)
- Lower respiratory airways that allow passage of atmospheric air into the lungs themselves – **main bronchi** and **bronchioles** (as conducting airways)
- Final respiratory airways that allow gaseous exchange to occur – **respiratory bronchioles, alveolar sacs** and **alveoli**

Unlike the cardiovascular system, which is sealed and enclosed, the respiratory system is open to the atmosphere to allow the intake of air during breathing.

During **inspiration** (breathing in), atmospheric air containing about 21% oxygen is drawn into and through the system via the nose or mouth, and down into the microscopic structure of the lungs to the **alveoli**.

It is here that some of the oxygen is exchanged with an accumulation of carbon dioxide gas, the waste product of the body cells' metabolic activities. The exchanged oxygen is taken away from the lungs in the circulatory system, to be used by the body during cellular activity, while the carbon dioxide is removed from the body during **expiration** (breathing out).

This **gaseous exchange mechanism** is the main function of the respiratory system.

THE THORACIC CAVITY – GROSS ANATOMY

The principal respiratory organs – the lungs – are situated in the **thorax** or chest cavity, one to the right of the **sternum** (the breast bone) and one to the left, with the heart lying over the latter's lower part.

Basic Guide to Anatomy and Physiology for Dental Care Professionals, First Edition. Carole Hollins.
© 2012 John Wiley & Sons, Ltd. Published 2012 by John Wiley & Sons, Ltd.

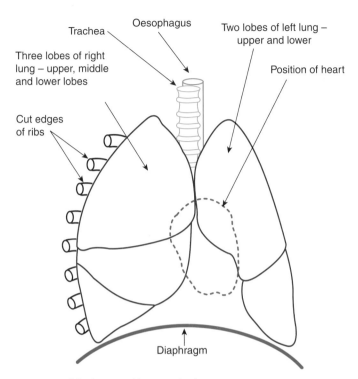

Figure 3.1 Position of the heart and lungs in the thorax.

The right lung has three lobes to its structure while the left lung has only two, due to the presence of the overlying heart.

The arrangement of the lungs and heart within the thorax is shown diagrammatically in Figure 3.1.

The thorax itself is an enclosed cavity composed of the thoracic spine behind, the rib cage and the sternum to the front.

The vertebrae of the spine articulate with the back of the rib cage, this cage then runs forwards and round to attach to the sternum. This creates the 'bell shape' of the chest cavity.

The base of this bell-shaped cavity is formed by a muscular sheet called the **diaphragm,** while the ribs are separated from each other by the **intercostal muscles.**

The movement of these **respiratory muscles** to increase the size of the chest cavity is instrumental in the respiratory process. The lungs themselves cannot increase their own size by inflation.

The inner surface of the thorax and the outer surface of the lungs are lined by the **pleural membranes,** which are separated by a thin layer of fluid that acts to lubricate the membranes during breathing movements.

The musculoskeletal anatomy of the thorax is illustrated in Figure 3.2.

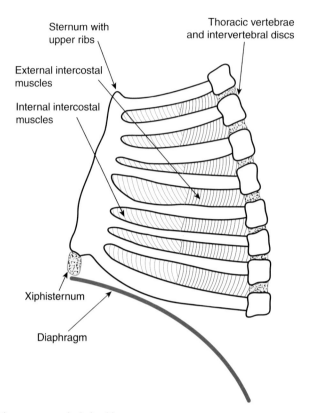

Figure 3.2 Thorax – musculoskeletal layout.

THE RESPIRATORY SYSTEM – GROSS ANATOMY

Air first enters the respiratory system through the nose, although in some situations it is also drawn in through the mouth. Mouth breathing tends to occur during exercise, when the body's demand for oxygen is increased, or in some people who tend to habitually breathe through their mouths.

Air passing through the nose tends to be warmed as it flows over the capillary network lining the nasal passages, and this makes it less irritant to the deeper structures of the system – inhaling cold air often stimulates coughing.

Inhaled air then passes to the back of the nose or mouth – the **pharynx,** and then to the **larynx** in the throat. The larynx forms the top end of the structure commonly called the windpipe, the **trachea,** and contains specialised flaps of tissue that form the **vocal cords.** The controlled movement of air over these cords form the speech sounds in humans.

In addition, the larynx contains a flap-like structure called the **epiglottis,** which falls across the top of the trachea during swallowing and so prevents food particles and fluids from entering the lungs.

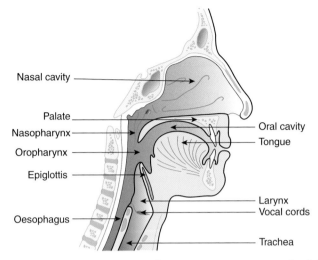

Nasal cavity

Palate

Nasopharynx

Oropharynx

Epiglottis

Oesophagus

Oral cavity

Tongue

Larynx
Vocal cords

Trachea

Figure 3.3 Upper respiratory tract. (From Hollins, C. (2008). *Levison's Textbook for Dental Nurses*, 10th edn. Blackwell Publishing, Oxford. Reproduced with permission from John Wiley & Sons, Ltd.)

RESPIRATORY SYSTEM

Up to this point, the anatomical structures of the respiratory system lie within the skull and the neck, but as the trachea approaches its lower end it enters the thoracic cavity.

The upper respiratory tract is shown in Figure 3.3.

The **trachea** and its two end branches, the right and left **bronchi**, are lined with rings of cartilage so that they form non-collapsible tubes. This ensures they remain open during breathing movements and allow the flow of inspired and expired air into and out of the lungs.

Each main bronchial tube then splits into two, and two again and again, to form the smaller conducting airways of the **bronchioles**, lying within the structure of the lungs themselves. Their function is simply to transport the inspired air to the deeper tissues of the lungs, warming and moistening it as it passes through.

The final branches of these conducting tubes, the **respiratory bronchioles**, are the points at which gaseous exchange first occurs. The airways continue to reduce in size until they run into the main structures concerned with respiration, the **alveolar sacs** containing the **alveoli**.

These microscopic structures provide a massive total surface area for gas exchange to occur, allowing the uptake of huge amounts of oxygen for body functions to continue.

UPPER RESPIRATORY TRACT – MICROSCOPIC ANATOMY

As stated previously, the nasal passages are the main entry port for inspired air, and they have a vast capillary network throughout their structure that helps to warm the air. In addition, the nostrils contain hairs that help to trap particulate debris such as dust specks, thereby preventing the entry of these larger foreign particles into the body.

Microscopically, the trachea and bronchi are lined by specialised epithelial cells that have hair-like projections called **cilia** over their surface. The cilia continually move in a wave-like motion and waft any smaller inhaled particles away from the lungs and towards the mouth, where they can be swallowed or spat out.

The inhaled particles will have become trapped first in a **mucus layer** secreted by goblet cells within the epithelium.

The walls of the trachea and bronchi contain rings and plates of cartilage so that they remain open during inspiration. Their diameters are therefore fixed and so contain little muscle in their structure.

LOWER RESPIRATORY TRACT – MICROSCOPIC ANATOMY

The bronchioles up to the alveolar sacs are surrounded by bundles of smooth muscle fibres, which allow these airways to alter their diameter as required – widening during exercise to increase the volume of air inspired, or narrowing to reduce the intake of noxious gases such as smoke.

This adjustment in size is called **bronchodilation** and **bronchoconstriction**, respectively.

In contrast to the upper airways, the bronchioles contain no cartilage and can therefore collapse when the air pressure within them is less than atmospheric pressure. This pressure difference can occur in situations such as during a prolonged or forced expiration.

ALVEOLI – MICROSCOPIC ANATOMY

The alveoli lie within the alveolar sacs at the very end of the respiratory system. They are composed of a thin layer of epithelial cells, often just one cell thick, and are surrounded by a huge network of **pulmonary capillaries**.

Some of the alveolar epithelial cells secrete fluid that lines the outside of the alveoli, allowing them to expand without any resistance during inspiration, as well as playing a key role in the gaseous exchange mechanism.

This microscopic, fluid-filled area is called the **interstitial space**.

Interspersed among the alveoli and capillaries is connective tissue, which holds the lung structure together and gives them their sponge-like appearance. This is called the **parenchyma**.

The microscopic anatomy of the alveoli is illustrated in Figure 3.4.

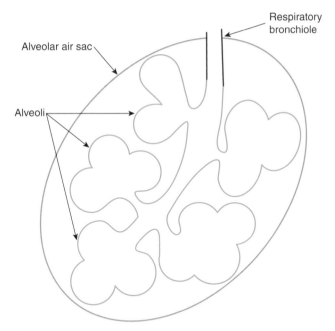

Respiratory
bronchiole

Alveolar air sac

Alveoli

Figure 3.4 Alveoli.

GASEOUS EXCHANGE MECHANISM

At rest, humans breathe at a rate of between 12 and 15 times per minute, and gaseous exchange between oxygen and carbon dioxide occurs during each of these breaths.

The pulmonary capillaries carry deoxygenated blood from the body to the lungs, via the pulmonary arteries. This blood contains a high concentration of carbon dioxide as the waste product of cell activity and metabolism, but little oxygen as this has been passed across to various body cells for use during the internal respiration process.

In contrast, the inspired air entering the alveoli contains a high concentration of oxygen but little carbon dioxide. Between the two areas then, there is a **concentration gradient** of these two gases, which allows the movement of them from one area to another.

By the laws of physics, all gases at different concentrations will tend to equilibrate themselves, by flowing from an area of high concentration to an area of low concentration, until the two areas are at an equal concentration.

So, **oxygen** dissolves into the fluid layer around the alveoli and then diffuses across the thin membrane between the air space and the surrounding capillaries, along the concentration gradient and into the pulmonary blood.

RESPIRATORY SYSTEM

Table 3.1 The proportions of oxygen and carbon dioxide in inspired and expired air.

	Oxygen	Carbon dioxide
Inspired air	21%	0.04%
Expired air	16%	4%

Once it reaches the blood plasma, it diffuses into the erythrocytes and binds itself to their haemoglobin molecules, ready to be transported to the body tissues as **oxyhaemoglobin**.

At the same time, **carbon dioxide** passes along its own concentration gradient by diffusing from the high concentration in the blood plasma of the pulmonary capillaries, as **bicarbonate ions**, across the air space and into the relatively low concentration within the alveoli.

It is then removed from the lungs during the next expiration.

The proportions of oxygen and carbon dioxide in inspired and expired air, which allows these concentration gradients to exist, are given in Table 3.1.

The transfer of these two gases in this way within the lungs is called **external respiration**.

The mechanism of external respiration is illustrated in Figure 3.5.

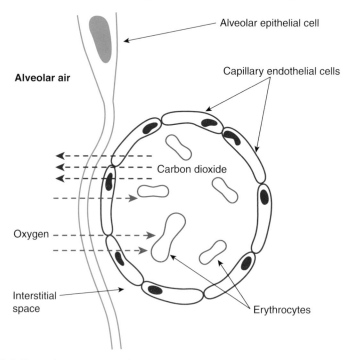

Figure 3.5 External respiration mechanism.

BREATHING MECHANISM

The lungs have no ability to expand and inflate themselves during respiration.

The breathing mechanism occurs entirely due to the movements of the thoracic cavity and the respiratory muscles, which are innervated by the **phrenic nerve,** the motor supply to the diaphragm, and the **intercostal nerves** providing the motor supply to the intercostal muscles.

Both sets of nerves are fired rhythmically by a group of specialised nerve cells within the brainstem, producing the subconscious action of rhythmic inspiration and expiration.

During inspiration, the volume of the thoracic cavity is increased, while it is decreased during expiration. The actions involved are as follows:

- Innervation of the phrenic nerve causes contraction of the diaphragm, which pulls it down from its usual dome shape just under the base of the lungs
- This muscle contraction increases the volume of the thoracic cavity, allowing the air pressure within the lungs to fall
- The pressure within the lungs is then less than that within the atmosphere, so air rushes from the higher to the lower pressure areas – that is, from the atmosphere into the lungs
- Inspiration occurs
- Expiration usually occurs as a passive event, due to the elastic recoil of the lungs and the chest wall, after having being stretched during inspiration
- When oxygen demands are increased (such as during exercise), the intercostal muscles contribute to both inspiratory and expiratory activity
- The chest volume is increased by these muscles lifting the rib cage upwards and out during inspiration
- The chest volume is decreased more rapidly during expiration by the contraction of the intercostal muscles

At rest, the volume of air inspired and expired with each breath is approximately 0.5 litres, and is called the **tidal volume.**

The total lung volume in an adult is up to 6 litres of air, and even during strenuous exercise this is not completely exchanged with the atmosphere – there is always a **residual volume** of about 1.2 litres of air, which is not exchanged during breathing but remains in the lungs.

In addition to the motor control of breathing, the diameter of the bronchioles themselves can be altered as required.

The smooth muscle of the bronchioles is activated by the **vagus nerve** (cranial nerve X) to cause bronchoconstriction, while bronchodilation occurs due to the effects of circulating **adrenaline** (epinephrine) in the pulmonary blood supply.

RESPIRATORY SYSTEM

Voluntary respiratory actions

Although the breathing mechanism itself is involuntary, the rate and depth of breathing can be consciously altered. The breathing rate can be increased by voluntarily **hyperventilating** (as occurs in controlled panting), although the similar hyperventilation that occurs during a panic attack is not voluntary.

Interestingly, during a panic attack the sufferer is expelling more carbon dioxide from the lungs than is being produced as a waste product by the body tissues. This has the adverse effect of altering the chemical composition and pH levels of the blood, causing the characteristic hyperventilation to occur.

Re-breathing expired air and its increased concentration of carbon dioxide (often with the aid of a paper bag), restores the chemical imbalance and reduces the respiratory rate, helping to calm the panicking subject.

When breathing is voluntarily suspended, by 'holding your breath', the length of time of the **voluntary apnoea** produced is controlled by the subsequent rise in carbon dioxide levels of the arterial blood. A point will be reached where the raised levels will stimulate the subject to breathe again involuntarily.

Chemical regulation and chemoreceptors

As indicated previously, even when the respiratory actions are altered voluntarily, the body will at some point overrule these actions and force the involuntary breathing mechanism to start again.

This involuntary mechanism relies on the body's response to the consequent varying levels of oxygen and carbon dioxide within the **arterial blood** supply that occurs during these events.

A chemical regulation mechanism exists that detects these disparities and activates the nerve supply involved with controlling the rate and depth of breathing movements. They are called **chemoreceptors**.

Those that lie outside the brain are called **peripheral chemoreceptors**, and those that lie within the brain are known as **central chemoreceptors**.

The peripheral chemoreceptors lie just at the point where the coronary arteries branch to form the internal and external carotid arteries, the main arterial supplies to the brain and the head.

These chemoreceptors are called the **carotid bodies** and are distinct anatomical structures that send nerve impulses to the brain when stimulated, via a branch of the **glossopharyngeal nerve** (cranial nerve IX).

Stimulation occurs when oxygen levels fall, carbon dioxide levels rise, or if the pH of the arterial blood passing through the carotid arteries alters.

In particular, the carotid bodies are responsible for altering the breathing mechanism in response to **hypoxia** – a situation that occurs when oxygen levels are too low for normal body requirements.

The central chemoreceptors respond specifically to pH changes in the **cerebrospinal fluid** of the central nervous system (the brain and spinal cord), rather than to changes within the arterial blood.

The pH changes occur as a direct result of raised carbon dioxide levels (a situation called **hypercapnia**), and these chemoreceptors are responsible for the majority of the chemical regulation of breathing under normal functioning conditions.

RESPIRATORY MEDICAL CONDITIONS

Asthma

This occurs as a result of exposure to an allergen, or as a response to exercise or exposure to cold climatic conditions.

During an asthma attack, the relevant stimulus causes the smooth muscle of the bronchi to go into spasm (**bronchospasm**), which results in a reduction in the diameter of these airways.

The sufferer experiences a distressing difficulty in breathing, known as **dyspnoea**, particularly when breathing out – indeed they can be seen to be quite clearly having to make a forced effort to exhale.

In acute cases, the sufferer can die if treatment to open the restricted airways is not given in time.

In chronic asthma, the bronchial epithelium is gradually destroyed so that the breathing mechanism becomes less efficient. The residual volume gradually elevates so that each inspiration provides less useable oxygen for the body tissues, until even minimal exercise will produce a state of hypoxia.

Pulmonary oedema

Although the alveoli are bathed externally by fluid lying in the interstitial space, the inner surface is dry in healthy individuals. Any excess fluid passing between the pulmonary capillaries and the interstitial space is normally removed by drainage into the pulmonary lymphatic system.

In situations where the fluid balance between these two areas fails, excess fluid will accumulate in the interstitial space and cause pulmonary oedema.

This occurs during **left-sided heart failure,** and as the situation worsens the excess fluid will flood into the alveoli themselves and prevent adequate gaseous exchange from occurring. Death will eventually result.

Bronchitis

Inflammation of the main bronchi occurs in two forms – either as **acute bronchitis,** of sudden onset and lasting just a few days, or **chronic bronchitis,** which is persistent and recurs over several years.

Acute bronchitis usually occurs as a complication of a viral infection (such as the common cold, or influenza), and is more prevalent in smokers and those with existing lung disease.

As the mucosal lining of the bronchi becomes inflamed, swelling and congestion occur and pus is formed. The sufferer experiences shortness of breath and wheezing, and has a persistent productive cough.

Repeated coughing often produces a 'ripping' pain behind the sternum, and the sufferer may be **pyrexic** (have a raised body temperature).

Chronic bronchitis is usually seen in smokers, or in those living in areas of high atmospheric pollution such as occurs in large industrialised cities.

Chronic irritation of the bronchi by these pollutants causes the overproduction of mucus by the lining epithelial cells.

The muscle layer of the bronchi and bronchioles thickens over time, narrowing their diameters and causing the natural removal of foreign particles to be less effective.

Infections are then more prone to occur and will cause further damage to the affected airways.

Emphysema

A disease caused by pollutant damage to the alveolar sacs and the alveoli themselves, resulting in their **distension** (abnormal widening). The main pollutant is tobacco smoke, although industrial pollutants also contribute to the damage caused.

The presence of these pollutants in inhaled air causes the alveoli to release chemicals that damage their walls and the lung parenchyma, and over time the damage can be so great that the alveoli eventually burst, and the lung structure loses its elasticity.

This gradually reduces the surface area available for gaseous exchange to occur, and oxygen levels in the blood will fall, resulting in dyspnoea and eventually **respiratory failure** or **right-sided heart failure**.

The resultant oxygen deficiency in the blood produces a blueness of the tissues to develop, called **cyanosis**.

COLD/COAD

When a sufferer has both chronic bronchitis and emphysema, they are said to be suffering from **chronic obstructive lung disease** (COLD), also called **chronic obstructive airways disease** (COAD).

Sufferers will experience a range of the symptoms associated with both disorders.

Cystic fibrosis

This is an inherited (genetic) disorder that results in reduced levels of fluid secretions by cells in the upper airway membranes. This allows the normal mucus produced to become abnormally thick and sticky, making its dislodgement and removal by the usual actions of the wafting cilia more difficult to achieve.

The smaller airways become restricted or even blocked with the mucus build-up, and sufferers experience repeated bronchial infections.

A strict, daily regime of physiotherapy exercises to dislodge the mucus and allow its removal by coughing and gravitational drainage is required to assist sufferers with the condition.

RESPIRATORY MEDICATIONS

Asthma

The aims of drug therapy are to reduce one of the following three causes of bronchial restriction associated with asthma:

- Bronchoconstriction
- Bronchial oedema
- Excessive mucus secretion

The majority of the drugs used to ease the symptoms of asthma can be inhaled, thereby acting directly on the airways affected:

- **Bronchodilators** – such as salbutamol inhalers, which are a compulsory component of the emergency drugs kit that must be held on every dental premise, and the drug theophylline
- **Corticosteroids** – such as beclomethasone inhalers, which help to reduce and control bronchial inflammation and oedema
- **Sodium cromoglycate** – as an inhaler, which works by blocking the release of histamine, thereby reducing mucus secretion

Pulmonary oedema

The aim of drug therapy is to reduce the fluid build-up in the lungs, so that gaseous exchange can occur:

- **Diuretics** – which reduce the fluid volume by increasing urine excretion by the kidneys, thereby increasing fluid output from the body
- **Bronchodilators** – such as aminophylline, which additionally acts to increase urine excretion by the kidneys, thereby aiding in fluid reduction too

Bronchitis

Acute bronchitis tends to resolve without any treatment other than a course of antibiotics, if the cause is bacterial.

The aims of drug therapy in cases of chronic bronchitis are to maximise the air intake to the lungs, and to prevent or treat any bronchial infections:

- **Bronchodilators** – given as an inhaler to relax and widen the bronchi, thereby allowing increased air flow to the lungs and reducing breathlessness
- **Expectorants** – to assist in the removal of accumulated sputum by coughing
- **Antibiotics** – to treat any bacterial lung infection, or prevent a bacterial infection developing in the first instance

Emphysema

The disease is incurable, so the aim of drug therapy is to control the symptoms experienced by the sufferer:

- **Bronchodilators** – as an inhaler or a nebuliser, to relax the bronchi and widen their diameter
- **Corticosteroids** – as an inhaler to reduce inflammation within the lungs
- **Diuretics** – to reduce the fluid volume of the body by increasing urine excretion, thereby relieving oedema
- **Oxygen therapy** – for sufferers experiencing hypoxia at rest, or showing signs of extensive cyanosis

Sufferers of COLD/COAD will have a combination of drug therapies to treat their bronchitis and/or emphysema symptoms, as required.

Cystic fibrosis

As the disease is genetic in origin, it cannot be prevented. Specialised physiotherapy techniques, aimed at draining the viscous mucus produced in the lungs of sufferers, is the most important daily requirement.

Drug therapy is aimed at treating any subsequent lung infection, by the use of specific **antibiotics.**

Chapter 4

Digestive system

The digestive system is composed of the following:

- The **mouth** and associated **salivary glands**
- The **pharynx**, where swallowing occurs
- The **oesophagus**, which transports food from the mouth to the stomach
- The **stomach**, where the majority of ingested foods are stored while being broken down for absorption
- The **small intestines**, where the final stages of digestion and absorption of various nutrients occurs
- The **large intestines**, where digestive waste products are stored before elimination, and water and salts are reabsorbed into the body
- Accessory digestive organs – the **pancreas, liver** and **gall bladder**

The mouth and the tongue, and in particular taste sensation, are covered in detail in Chapter 7, while the salivary glands are covered in Chapter 10.

The digestive system, or **gastrointestinal tract** (GI tract) as it is correctly termed, is effectively an open hollow tube running from the mouth to the anus, with various specialised sections along its way that are involved in food digestion.

The foods acted upon are carbohydrates, proteins and fats.

The pharynx lies at the back of the mouth and into the throat, while the oesophagus runs through the thoracic cavity and connects to all other parts of the GI tract, which lie in the abdominal cavity and beneath the diaphragm.

The GI tract and the accessory digestive organs are illustrated in Figure 4.1.

THE PHARYNX – GROSS ANATOMY

Food enters the GI tract in the mouth, where it is chewed (**masticated**) into smaller portions to form a bolus, and then mixed with saliva before being swallowed.

Basic Guide to Anatomy and Physiology for Dental Care Professionals, First Edition. Carole Hollins.
© 2012 John Wiley & Sons, Ltd. Published 2012 by John Wiley & Sons, Ltd.

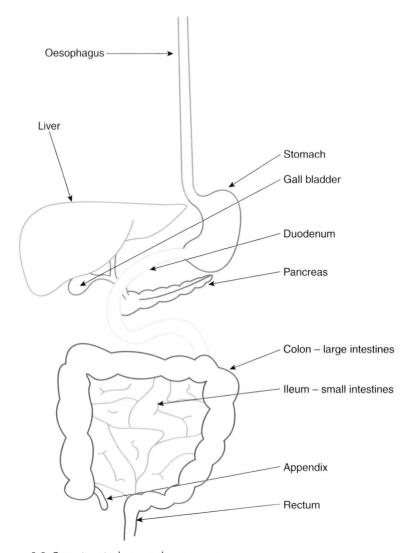

Figure 4.1 Gastrointestinal tract and accessory organs.

Voluntary tongue actions move the bolus towards the back of the mouth, the **oropharynx**, and then into the **laryngopharynx** of the throat. This region forms the topmost opening of both the oesophagus and the trachea, with the trachea lying in front of the oesophagus in the neck.

A flap of cartilage called the **epiglottis** projects from the front wall of the larynx, and is instrumental in preventing food and fluids from entering the topmost opening of the trachea, the **glottis**, during swallowing.

The oropharynx also communicates with the nasal passages at an area behind the **soft palate** called the **nasopharynx**.

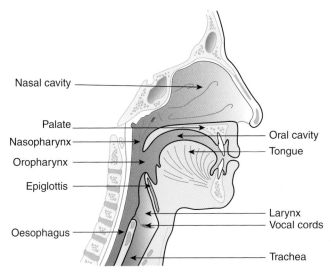

Figure 4.2 Pharynx and larynx. (From Hollins, C. (2008). *Levison's Textbook for Dental Nurses*, 10th edn. Blackwell Publishing, Oxford. Reproduced with permission from John Wiley & Sons, Ltd.)

The anatomy of the pharynx and larynx is illustrated in Figure 4.2.

Swallowing

The act of swallowing a bolus of masticated food or a fluid is both a voluntary and involuntary action. The medical term for swallowing is **deglutition**.

Initially, the food bolus is directed voluntarily towards the oropharynx by the muscular actions of the tongue. This is known as the **oral phase** of swallowing.

The tongue shapes the bolus into a circular or 'sausage-shaped' mass, using its flexible tip and rolled sides to press the bolus into shape against the roof of the mouth – the **hard palate**, before guiding it posteriorly.

At this point, the involuntary **pharyngeal phase** begins.

The soft palate rises to seal off the nasal passages, while a coordinated muscular contractile wave propels the bolus through the relaxed oesophageal opening (the **oesophageal sphincter**) and into the oesophagus itself.

The muscular wave is called **peristalsis** and occurs throughout the length of the GI tract, moving the food bolus in one direction only.

At the same time, the larynx is raised to close the glottis and the epiglottis falls across it so that respiration is temporarily stopped. This prevents the food bolus from falling into the trachea and being inhaled into the lungs.

Once the bolus enters the oesophagus, the final involuntary **oesophageal phase** of swallowing occurs. Peristalsis continues to move the bolus along the length of the oesophagus and into the stomach, taking just up to 10 seconds to do so. Fluids pass much more quickly.

The junction of the oesophagus and the stomach – the **cardiac sphincter** – relaxes as the peristaltic wave approaches, and the bolus is allowed to enter the stomach itself.

Once the bolus has entered the stomach, the sphincter contracts and tightens again so that food contents cannot reflux back into the oesophagus under normal circumstances.

The swallowing sequence is illustrated in Figure 4.3.

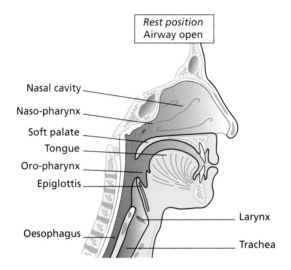

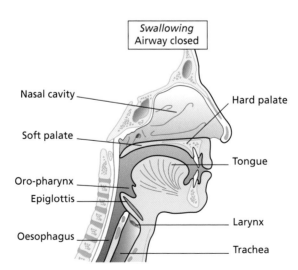

Figure 4.3 Swallowing sequence. (From Hollins, C. (2008). *Levison's Textbook for Dental Nurses*, 10th edn. Blackwell Publishing, Oxford. Reproduced with permission from John Wiley & Sons, Ltd.)

DIGESTIVE SYSTEM

THE STOMACH – GROSS ANATOMY

The stomach lies in the upper left quadrant of the abdominal cavity, just below the diaphragm. It connects at the top end to the oesophagus at the cardiac sphincter, and at its lower end to the small intestines at the **pyloric sphincter.**

Other than the initialisation of carbohydrate digestion that occurs in the mouth, the stomach is the organ where the breakdown and digestion of food truly begins.

Consequently, it has an extensive blood supply from the **gastric arteries,** which branch repeatedly to form a vascular network around the organ. All the blood supplied to the stomach leaves the organ via the gastric veins, which drain into the **portal vein** supplying the liver. This arrangement ensures that all ingested products pass through the liver for further chemical processing, before the blood joins the main circulation again.

The stomach has several functions, as follows:

- Storage of food when it first enters the digestive tract
- Mechanical food breakdown, to form **chyme**
- Digestion of **proteins**
- Production of **gastric acid**
- Transport of chyme to the small intestines, for further digestion

THE STOMACH – MICROSCOPIC ANATOMY

In general with the microscopic anatomy of most areas of the GI tract, the stomach is composed of the following basic structures:

- Outer wall called the **serosa,** made up of epithelium and connective tissue, which is continuous with that lining the abdominal cavity, and holds the abdominal contents in place
- Outer **longitudinal smooth muscle** layer, which contracts in synchrony to help propel the GI tract contents along its length
- Inner **circular smooth muscle** layer, which also contracts in synchrony so that peristalsis movement occurs
- Thickened areas of circular smooth muscle form the cardiac and pyloric sphincters, at either end of the stomach
- A third layer of muscle, unique to the stomach and called the **oblique smooth muscle** layer, which allows the organ to carry out churning movements to help break down food particles and aid digestion
- A **submucosal** layer of connective tissue, blood vessels and lymphatic drainage vessels
- An inner **mucosal** layer, containing various specialised cells

Specialised cells of the gastric mucosa

With these mucous cells, the other cells making up the gastric mucosa occur in specialised regions called **gastric glands**, and consist of the following:

- **Mucous cells** – which secrete alkaline mucus
- **Chief cells** – which secrete inactive **pepsinogen**
- **Parietal cells** – which secrete **hydrochloric acid** and **intrinsic factor**
- **G cells** – which secrete the hormone **gastrin**

A gastric gland is illustrated in Figure 4.4.

The various functions of these cells and their gastric secretions are summarised in the following text.

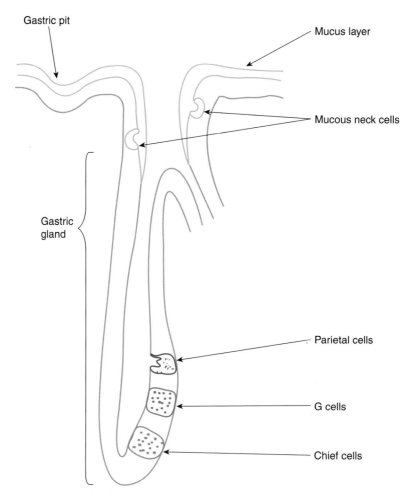

Figure 4.4 Gastric gland.

Mucous cells

- Form the majority of the surface cells of the stomach mucosa
- Secrete an **alkaline mucus**
- This forms a protective lining over the inner surface of the organ and acts to prevent self-digestion in an otherwise very acidic environment

Chief cells

- Lie deep within the gastric glands
- Secrete **pepsinogen,** an inactive form of the enzyme pepsin
- **Pepsin** breaks down protein foodstuffs

Parietal cells

- Lie scattered throughout the gastric glands
- Secrete **hydrochloric acid** when stimulated by food ingestion
- This produces an acidic environment of pH 2 within the stomach
- The low pH kills many ingested micro-organisms, such as salmonella
- It helps to break down meaty foods
- It converts pepsinogen to the active enzyme pepsin, for protein digestion
- Also secrete **intrinsic factor,** which is essential for the absorption of **vitamin B12** (required for the production of erythrocytes)

G cells

- Lie close to the chief cells
- Secrete the hormone **gastrin** into the bloodstream
- Gastrin stimulates the parietal cells to release hydrochloric acid, until the stomach pH falls below 3
- It also stimulates the release of enzymes and mucus

The cells of the gastric glands only produce their various secretions when stimulated. The main initial stimulation occurs in response to the anticipation of having a meal – the sight, smell and taste of food, as well as its presence within the mouth before swallowing.

Appetite-regulating areas of the brain are activated and send signals to the stomach via the **vagus nerve** (cranial nerve X) once the food is swallowed and enters the organ.

This has the following effects:

- Directly increases gastric acid secretion by acting on the parietal cells
- Indirectly increases gastric acid secretion by acting on G cells to release gastrin

DIGESTIVE SYSTEM

As peristalsis moves the partially digested food from the stomach to the small intestines, G cells here are stimulated to release more gastrin for a short time, so that digestion continues.

Very little absorption of food occurs in the stomach, except for alcohol, and no water at all is absorbed.

VOMITING

This is a protective mechanism that acts to quickly and forcefully expel noxious and toxic substances from the GI tract, before damage is caused. It is controlled in a specialised area of the brain, called the **medulla**, and may occur due to other stimuli, such as the following, rather than as a protective mechanism:

- Pain
- Hormonal imbalance (such as 'morning sickness')
- Some drugs and anaesthetic gases
- Emotional response to unpleasant sights or smells
- Radiation overexposure ('radiation sickness')
- Disturbances with spatial awareness (such as labyrinthitis, motion sickness and vertigo)

THE SMALL INTESTINES – GROSS ANATOMY

The small intestines are connected to the end of the stomach at the pyloric sphincter, and have three distinct sections to them:

- **Duodenum**
- **Jejunum**
- **Ileum**

They connect to the large intestines at the end of the ileum.

The final stages of digestion and the absorption of some nutrients occur in the small intestines.

The chyme produced in the stomach passes into the duodenum and is mixed with **pancreatic juice** and **bile**, which has been stored in the gall bladder after being made by the liver.

THE SMALL INTESTINES – MICROSCOPIC ANATOMY

As with the stomach, the small intestines are very well adapted to carry out their digestive and absorptive functions, not only by cellular specialisations but by their huge surface area too.

The internal surface area is massively increased by the presence of finger-like projections called **villi** throughout the length of the small intestines. The mucosal covering of the epithelial cells forming the villi are also covered in tiny projections called **microvilli**, which increases the surface area available for absorption even further.

The intestinal surface itself is arranged into **circular folds**, which causes the chyme to flow through in a slowed spiral motion, thereby increasing the time available for nutritional absorption to occur.

Beneath the surface of each villus are a dense capillary network and a lymph vessel, so that absorbed nutrients are transported easily to the liver in the portal vein, and absorbed water is removed quickly from the area via the lymphatic system.

The microscopic anatomy of the small intestine is illustrated in Figure 4.5.

The specialised cells within the small intestines are concerned with secreting alkaline fluids and mucus, to help neutralise the acidity of the chyme leaving the stomach. The digestion that occurs within the small intestines is due to pancreatic and bile secretions.

THE LARGE INTESTINES – GROSS ANATOMY

The large intestines are connected to the end of the ileum at the **ileocaecal valve**, and anatomically they are divided into four sections:

- Caecum
- Colon
- Rectum
- Anal canal

The caecum is a pouch-like structure that is separated from the ileum by a flap of mucosa, the ileocaecal valve. This acts as a one-way valve and prevents the regurgitation of the GI tract contents back into the small intestines, once they have passed into the caecum.

Both the caecum and the attached structure called the **appendix**, forming this first section of the large intestines, have no digestive function in humans.

The colon constitutes the main section of the large intestines, and runs up, across and down the abdominal cavity, joining the rectum at the final section called the **sigmoid colon**.

It receives blood via the **mesenteric arteries**, and is drained via the mesenteric veins into the **hepatic portal vein**.

The final parts of the large intestines are made up of the rectum and the anal canal, and are involved in the expulsion of the GI tract waste products by defaecation.

Intestinal wall layers

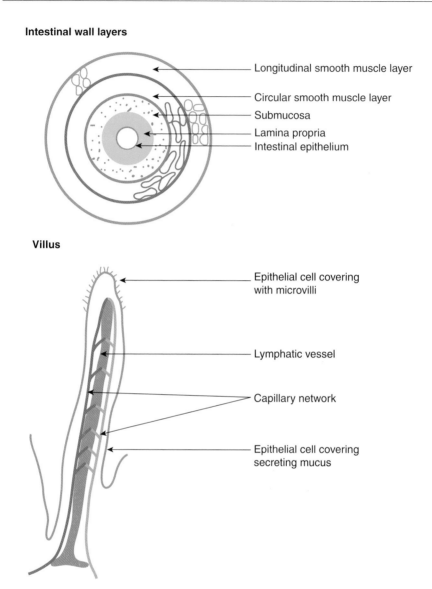

Longitudinal smooth muscle layer

Circular smooth muscle layer

Submucosa

Lamina propria

Intestinal epithelium

Villus

Epithelial cell covering
with microvilli

Lymphatic vessel

Capillary network

Epithelial cell covering
secreting mucus

Figure 4.5 Layers of intestinal wall and a villus.

The anal canal and the anus form the end section of the GI tract.

The digestive role of the GI tract is completed in the small intestines, so the main functions of the large intestines, especially the colon, are:

- Storage of the resultant semi-solid mass of food residue, until it is eliminated from the body as faeces
- Absorption of water and electrolytes from this residue, back into the body to prevent dehydration

- Secretion of mucus, to allow the smooth passage of the resultant waste mass
- Fermentation of any indigestible carbohydrates and fats, making their passage and removal from the body possible
- Accommodation of various intestinal bacteria, which help to break down some drugs, and to synthesise various dietary vitamins (vitamin K and some of the B vitamins)

THE LARGE INTESTINES – MICROSCOPIC ANATOMY

As no digestion occurs in the large intestines, the microscopic anatomy of the region is much simpler in nature.

There are no villi present, nor specialised cells involved with digestion; indeed, the main component of the large intestines is various layers of muscle.

The microscopic anatomy is as follows:

- Outer wall of connective tissue that attaches the large intestines to the inner lining of the abdominal cavity, the **peritoneum**
- Outer layer of **longitudinal smooth muscle,** which lies in three bands and pulls the colon section into pouches
- This enables the large intestines to store various amounts of waste products before elimination
- Thick inner **circular smooth muscle** layer
- The muscle layers act together to continue the movement of the GI tract contents towards the anus, via peristalsis
- **Submucosal layer** of connective tissue and blood vessels
- Inner **mucosal layer** made up of large numbers of **intestinal glands**
- These are lined with **epithelial absorptive cells** and mucus secreting **goblet cells**

ACCESSORY DIGESTIVE ORGANS

The pancreas – gross anatomy

The pancreas lies across the upper abdomen, partially behind the stomach and with its 'head' lying in a curve of the duodenum (see Figure 4.1).

Its main duct is connected to the duodenum at the **duodenal papilla,** just at the point where the bile duct from the gall bladder also joins the GI tract.

The pancreas is essentially a glandular organ, and has a rich blood supply via the **mesenteric arteries.** Its venous blood is taken directly to the liver via the **portal vein.**

DIGESTIVE SYSTEM

The functions of the pancreas are as follows:

- **Endocrine gland** – secreting **hormones** directly into the circulatory system
  - **Insulin** – to promote the absorption of glucose from the blood, and into the liver and muscle cells for storage
  - **Glucagon** – to promote the release of the stored glucose from the liver and the muscle cells, for use by the body tissues
- So the two hormones work against each other to control the blood glucose levels in the body and maintain them within a narrow range
- **Exocrine gland** – secreting **enzymes** into the GI tract at the duodenum to assist the breakdown of food substances during digestion

The pancreas – microscopic anatomy

The pancreas is shaped like a carrot, with a thick 'head' end that narrows to a thinner 'tail' end, with the **pancreatic duct** running along the full length of the organ.

The pancreatic tissue is arranged in lobules, with the vast majority of it making up the exocrine portion of the gland, while the tissue forming the endocrine portion is scattered throughout this as isolated clumps of specialised tissue called the **islets of Langerhans**.

The exocrine tissue is arranged as balls of secretory cells surrounding a central space, into which their digestive enzymes are discharged. The balls of tissue are called **acini**, and their secretory ducts channel the fluid discharge into ever-widening passages, until they all empty their contents into the pancreatic duct.

The ducts are lined with epithelial cells that secrete **pancreatic juice**, and the mixture of juice and enzymes flow towards the duodenum to aid digestion.

Just before the pancreatic duct joins the duodenum, it fuses with the common bile duct from the gall bladder at a specialised area of tissue called the **sphincter of Oddi**.

The sphincter controls the release of both bile and pancreatic juice into the duodenum.

The structure of the acini is illustrated in Figure 4.6.

Digestive role of pancreatic juice and bile

The juices these organs release are alkaline, and therefore contribute to the neutralisation of the acidic chyme as it leaves the stomach. This prevents any corrosive effects on the inner surface of the small intestines.

The pancreas in particular plays a huge role in digestion, by releasing many different enzymes or their inactive precursors to break down various food substances. The main ones are as follows:

- **Trypsin** – released as inactive **trypsinogen** and responsible for protein digestion

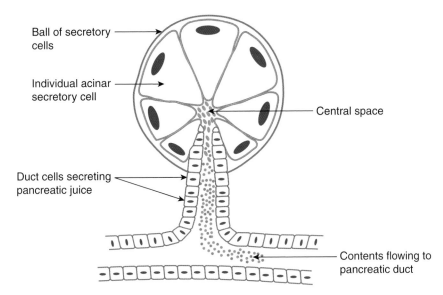

Figure 4.6 Pancreatic acini.

- **Amylase** – released direct, and responsible for the completion of the carbohydrate digestion that began in the mouth
- **Lipase** – released direct, and responsible for fat digestion

Bile is mainly involved in neutralising the acidic chyme that leaves the stomach, and in emulsifying fats to aid their digestion.

The end products of digestion, the nutrients that are required for the cells of the body to work, pass from the lumen of the small intestines into the surrounding capillaries in a similar fashion to the movement of gases during external and internal respiration (see Chapter 3).

The nutrients produced from each food product are as follows:

- **Carbohydrates** are broken down into simple sugars – such as **glucose** and **fructose**
- **Proteins** are broken down into **peptides** and **amino acids**
- **Fats** are broken down into **fatty acids** and **glycerol**

In addition, vitamins, water and electrolytes (such as sodium, iron and calcium) are absorbed at various points in the GI tract, although mainly in the small intestines.

The GI tract plays a very important role in regulating the fluid and electrolyte balance of the body, as excessive loss of either would result in dehydration and metabolic imbalance – both of which can lead to death in severe cases.

Endocrine functions of the pancreas

The cells within the endocrine portion of the pancreas – the islets of Langerhans – are mainly of two types:

- **Alpha cells** – make and secrete **glucagon,** which acts to release stored glucose from body cells into the bloodstream
- The main stimulus for the release of glucagon is the condition of low blood glucose – **hypoglycaemia**
- **Beta cells** – make and secrete **insulin,** which acts to promote the uptake of glucose from the blood to be stored in the body tissues
- The main stimulus for insulin secretion is a rise in blood glucose levels – **hyperglycaemia**

The liver – gross anatomy

The liver is the largest organ in the body, and lies in the top right corner of the abdominal cavity, just beneath the diaphragm (see Figure 4.1).

It is composed of two large lobes (small left and larger right), with two much smaller lobes lying on the back surface of the right lobe. The **gall bladder** is also situated here.

The liver has many metabolic functions, and receives not only its own blood supply via the **hepatic artery,** but it also receives blood rich in nutrients from the GI tract via the **hepatic portal vein.**

All of the blood arriving via the hepatic portal vein therefore passes through the liver itself, before returning to the systemic circulation through the hepatic vein and into the **inferior vena cava.**

The functions of the liver are as follows:

- **Carbohydrate metabolism** – the body's main reserve of carbohydrate is stored as glycogen in the liver, and is available for release into the blood stream on demand. The liver can also form **glucose** by the digestion of carbohydrate
- **Fat metabolism** – fats are not water soluble, so they cannot be absorbed directly from the GI tract as other nutrients are. Instead, they are absorbed by the liver, along with fat-soluble vitamins
- **Bile production** – bile allows fats to be **emulsified** (broken down into droplets in solution) so that they can be absorbed by the liver
- **Protein synthesis** – the liver manufactures many plasma proteins, including albumin and the **clotting factor proteins,** which are necessary for the process of blood clotting
- **Storage** – the liver is responsible for the storage of both **iron** and **vitamin B12,** which are essential for the formation of erythrocytes
- **Detoxification** – the vast majority of ingested drugs and toxins (such as alcohol) are detoxified ('made safe') in the liver before being excreted
- **Endocrine function** – various hormones are manufactured in the liver

The liver – microscopic anatomy

Each lobe of the liver is made up of irregularly shaped **lobules** with a central vein emptying into the hepatic vein. Around the outer borders of the lobules are structures called **portal triads** – a bundle of three vessels, functioning as follows:

- **Branch of hepatic artery** – providing oxygenated blood to the liver tissue itself
- **Branch of hepatic portal vein** – supplying nutrient-rich blood directly from the GI tract
- **Branch of bile duct** – transporting the bile made within the liver to the duodenum for fat absorption, or to the gall bladder for storage

The lobules themselves are made up of liver cells, known as **hepatocytes,** which are loosely arranged around the central vein to form the spongy tissue of the liver.

They are bathed in the blood from both supplies running in the portal triads, and allow the free transfer of fluid between the blood plasma and the lobules. Excess fluid within the lobules drains into lymphatic vessels, and is removed from the organ.

A liver lobule is illustrated in Figure 4.7.

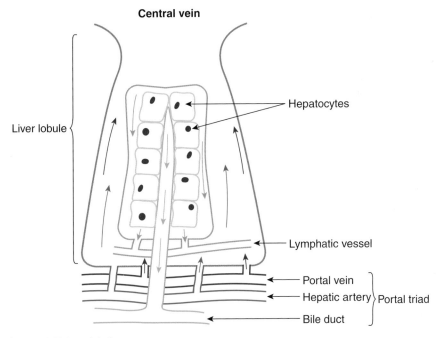

Figure 4.7 Liver lobule.

DIGESTIVE SYSTEM

The role of the gall bladder

The gall bladder is a muscular sac lying behind the right lobe of the liver, and connected to the pancreatic duct at the sphincter of Oddi.

Bile produced by the hepatocytes in the liver is transported along the bile ducts to the gall bladder for storage. The bile becomes more concentrated with time, as water and electrolytes are reabsorbed by the gall bladder, leaving bile salts and bile pigments as its main constituents.

The bile salts are made in the liver from cholesterol, and are essential in the processing of dietary fats in the duodenum.

Bile pigments are the end products of erythrocyte breakdown in the spleen, the main pigment being **bilirubin**. The pigments are excreted as waste products in faeces.

The release of bile from the gall bladder is stimulated by the eating of a meal, especially one rich in fats. The bile salts act on the fat globules in the chyme by emulsification, breaking them down into small droplets suspended in solution.

In this form, they can be absorbed from the portal vein blood into the liver, and then broken down during digestion for use by the body tissues.

GASTROINTESTINAL MEDICAL CONDITIONS

Dysphagia

Difficulty in swallowing (**dysphagia**) is usually due to an actual underlying medical condition, including any of the following:

- Dry mouth (**xerostomia**)
- Mucosal damage due to acid reflux conditions
- Poor muscular control during swallowing
- Oesophageal tightening, due to scarring from reflux, or from oesophageal tumours
- Poor nervous control during swallowing, due to a stroke or other central nervous conditions

It does not tend to refer to the intermittent inability to swallow due to psychological reasons, as can occur when taking medicinal tablets for instance. Sufferers of this condition are always able to swallow food products, but experience an inability to swallow medicinal solids.

Gastro-oesophageal reflux

This occurs when the stomach contents pass back (**reflux**) into the oesophagus, and results from an increased abdominal pressure over the thoracic pressure,

DIGESTIVE SYSTEM

or when the cardiac sphincter of the stomach remains relaxed for extensive periods.

The pressure difference often occurs in the following instances:

- After a heavy meal
- Particularly if eaten just before lying down or bending
- In the late stages of pregnancy, when the size of the foetus displaces the other abdominal contents

The burning sensation of the acidic stomach contents in the oesophagus causes the typical pain of **indigestion** or 'heartburn'.

In severe instances, this can be mistaken for the pain associated with angina, or even a heart attack.

Hiatus hernia

The oesophagus passes through the diaphragm to join the stomach in the abdominal cavity at a natural opening called the **hiatus**.

When a hiatus hernia occurs, the junction of the oesophagus and the stomach moves up through the opening in the diaphragm and becomes trapped there, so that a portion of the stomach is lying above the diaphragm itself.

This restricts the normal digestive movements and emptying of the stomach, and causes a reflux of stomach contents into the oesophagus. Again, the pain of indigestion will be felt by hernia sufferers, especially after a meal has been taken.

Hiatus hernias usually require surgical intervention to repair the diaphragm.

Gastric ulcers

During normal function, the stomach protects itself from acid damage by producing a protective layer of mucus and alkaline fluid from its specialised cells, and by preventing acid leakage into the submucosa by having tight junctions between the epithelial cells.

Any drug or condition that increases acid production, or slows down mucus production, may allow acid leakage into the submucosa and result in inflammation of the inner lining of the stomach – **gastritis**.

When severe enough, the submucosa is eroded and an ulcer develops.

Drugs and conditions associated with gastric (and duodenal) ulcers are:

- **Caffeine,** especially from strong coffee
- **Nicotine**
- **Non-steroidal anti-inflammatory drugs** (NSAIDs) such as aspirin and ibuprofen
- **Stress**
- Infection with *Helicobacter pylori* within the stomach itself

Coeliac disease

This is a disorder of absorption affecting the small intestines, in which there is an intolerance to **gluten**.

Gluten is a cereal protein found particularly in wheat, rye, oats and barley, and when these products are eaten a hypersensitivity response occurs. The chemical composition of gluten mimics that of an immune complex that promotes an immune response within the small intestines.

The toxins produced during the immune response damage the lining of the small intestines; in particular, they gradually destroy the villi.

The sufferer is then unable to absorb nutrients from food as it passes through the small intestines, and obvious weight loss and general malaise occur.

Once diagnosed and started on a gluten-free diet, the health of the sufferer should improve rapidly and be maintained as long as the specialised diet is followed – therefore, it must be for life.

Crohn's disease

A chronic inflammatory disease that can affect any part of the GI tract (including the mouth, as recurrent apthous ulcers), but which usually occurs in the ileum, particularly at its end where it joins the large intestines.

The cause is unknown, but it may be an allergic reaction to an infectious agent. With time, the walls of the intestines become thickened and its ability to absorb nutrients from food diminishes, so that the sufferer becomes generally unwell and loses weight.

In severe cases, the intestinal swelling is bad enough to restrict normal peristalsis, and GI tract obstructions occur. Abscesses and fistulas (abnormal passageways) also occur in a significant number of sufferers.

In severe cases, surgery may be required to remove sections of the GI tract that have become badly diseased or obstructed.

Ulcerative colitis

A chronic inflammatory disease that affects the lining of the colon and rectum only, rather than affecting any section of the GI tract, as does Crohn's disease.

Its cause is unknown, and symptoms tend to be more severe than with Crohn's disease. Anaemia may occur due to extensive blood loss from the ulcerated colon, and in long-standing cases there is an increased risk of developing bowel cancer.

In severe cases, and at the first indication of cancer, the colon may have to be surgically removed – a procedure called **colectomy**.

DIGESTIVE SYSTEM

Diverticular disease

The blood vessels supplying the colon have to penetrate the thick circular smooth muscle layer of its structure, to allow the water reabsorbed from the semi-solid food waste material to enter the circulatory system and be transported to the hepatic portal vein.

These areas of penetration are potential weak points in the colon wall, and pressure within the colon can force its own lining through these weak points (herniate) to protrude externally as pouches, or **diverticulae**.

It is thought that a diet low in fibre may increase the risk of developing diverticular disease.

When the pouches are present, the sufferer has **diverticulosis**, but when they become inflamed due to rupture, the sufferer has **diverticulitis**.

If symptoms occur with diverticulosis, a dietary change to increase fibre intake usually improves the situation, and other treatment is often not necessary.

Irritable bowel syndrome

A common condition in which sufferers have a combination of intermittent abdominal pain and irregular bowel habits – bouts of constipation and/or diarrhoea. It is said to be present when these symptoms occur in the absence of any other diagnosed GI tract disease.

The cause is unknown, although its occurrence tends to be stress related. Symptoms can be eased considerably by starting a diet high in fibre.

Chronic pancreatitis

Inflammation of the pancreas may be acute or chronic, but the latter condition is more serious as it results in permanent damage to the pancreas. The scar tissue formed gradually reduces the efficiency of the pancreas in releasing its digestive enzymes, resulting in **malabsorption** of the sufferer, as they are unable to adequately digest nutrients from food.

If the damaged region of the organ involves the islets of Langerhans, the sufferer will develop **diabetes** due to the resultant insufficient production of insulin.

The cause is most often related to excessive alcohol intake, although the presence of gallstones at the exit of the pancreatic duct, causing its blockage, will also cause pancreatitis.

The vast majority of cystic fibrosis sufferers also exhibit inadequate pancreatic function, as part of their genetic condition.

Diabetes mellitus

This is a disorder caused by a reduced or non-existent production of insulin by the pancreas.

There are two types of diabetes:

- **Type I insulin-dependent diabetes** – the more severe form, and developing in younger sufferers, it occurs rapidly following the destruction of the islets tissue as an immune response, often following a viral infection
- **Type II non-insulin-dependent diabetes** – develops gradually in older sufferers, and is the result of insufficient insulin production, there is often a genetic predisposition to the disease

The reduced, or absent, levels of insulin allow a rise in blood glucose levels, which produce the following symptoms to a greater or lesser degree:

- **Excess urine production** – as the body attempts to eliminate the glucose, as it cannot be stored or used by the body tissues
- **Excessive thirst** – as a result of the increased loss of fluid from the body by urination
- **Prone to infection** – as the excess glucose levels impair the ability of the body cells to fight infection
- **Weight loss** – as the body cells release stored fat in an attempt to generate some energy
- **Fatigue** – as the body cells are unable to take up and use the circulating glucose for energy production
- **Peripheral neuropathy** – tingling and numbness in the extremities, as peripheral nerves and blood vessels degenerate more rapidly

Many Type II diabetics are unaware of their disorder, although obesity is the main factor that generates medical intervention and a diagnosis.

Sensible dietary measures combined with controlled weight reduction are often all that many Type II diabetics require to keep their symptoms under control.

Hepatitis

Inflammation of the liver can be related to alcohol abuse, other poisons, drug overdose or due to a viral infection.

The relevant viral infections are classified as **Hepatitis A, B or C**, with Hepatitis B being of particular concern in dentistry as it is blood borne.

All clinical dental personnel are therefore required to be vaccinated against Hepatitis B throughout their clinical working lives.

The sufferer experiences flu-like symptoms and will exhibit **jaundice**, the unnatural yellow discolouration of the skin and the whites of the eyes associated with a build-up of the bile pigment **bilirubin**.

Avoidance by vaccination is the obvious course of action with viral infections, and abstinence from alcohol or other poisons will allow the liver to repair and regenerate itself over time otherwise.

Where the damage is severe enough to result in **liver failure** (the loss of liver function), a liver transplant will ultimately be required to save the patient's life.

Gallstones

These develop as solid lumps ('stones') in the gall bladder, due to a disruption in the chemical composition of bile.

The disruption is usually due to an increase in **cholesterol** content of the bile, as occurs in obese sufferers, or due to a lack of emulsifying agents that normally keep the cholesterol in solution.

If the stones block the bile ducts, the sufferer will experience severe pain and usually will require the surgical removal of the gall bladder.

Where symptoms are not experienced, no treatment is required, or the stones can be shattered with a special ultrasound device that allows the fragments to pass naturally from the body via the GI tract.

GASTROINTESTINAL MEDICATIONS

Gastro-oesophageal reflux

Avoidance of eating large meals, especially just before bed or taking exercise will prevent many instances of reflux.

In other cases, the aim of drug therapy is to neutralise the gastric acid that has entered the oesophagus and caused the pain of indigestion:

- **Antacids** – often available as 'over-the-counter' remedies, and contain neutralising agents such as sodium bicarbonate and magnesium hydroxide
- **Acid production suppressants** – such as omeprazole, which act to prevent the release of acid from the parietal cells of the stomach

Gastric ulcers

The reduction or avoidance of the drugs associated with ulcer formation is the ideal action to take, thereby preventing their formation in the future.

The aim of drug therapy is to reduce the acid production of the stomach and heal the ulcerated areas:

- **Acid production suppressants** – such as omeprazole, which act to prevent the release of acid from the parietal cells
- **Ulcer-healing drugs** – such as cimetidine and ranitidine, which block the actions of histamine on the parietal cells, thereby reducing acid secretion

Crohn's disease and ulcerative colitis

The aim of drug therapy is to limit the inflammatory damage to the ileum or the colon:

- **Corticosteroids** – which act to reduce the inflammation, and are given in short, intense courses to avoid the suppression of the adrenal glands to release corticosteroids naturally
- **Sulphasalazine** – which acts to prevent inflammation from developing generally

Chronic pancreatitis

The aim of drug therapy is to replace the pancreatic enzymes that are no longer produced due to the damage to the pancreas:

- **Pancreatin** – a combination of pancreatic digestive enzymes given as a supplement, to allow normal digestion to proceed

Diabetes mellitus

In Type II diabetes, dietary control alone is often sufficient in stabilising blood glucose levels, especially by controlling carbohydrate intake.

The aim of drug therapy is to allow the body to control the blood glucose levels accurately:

- **Insulin injections** – for Type I diabetics, self-injected as a predetermined dose before meals to allow glucose uptake to occur, thereby reducing the blood glucose levels
- **Oral hypoglycaemics** – such as tolbutamide for Type II diabetics, which act by increasing insulin production in the pancreas so that glucose uptake from the blood to the body cells can occur

Chapter 5

Nervous system

The nervous system is composed of the following:

- The **brain** and **spinal cord**, forming the **central nervous system**
- The **peripheral nerves, autonomic nerves** and **enteric nerves,** forming the **peripheral nervous system**
- The sensory organs of the **eyes,** the **ears,** the **tongue (taste)** and the **nose (smell)**

The tongue and taste sensation are covered in detail in Chapter 7.

Details of the other sensory organs are beyond the remit of this text.

The brain is the organ responsible for the continuation of life for all organisms, by acting as the control centre of the body. All basic life functions, such as maintenance of the heart rate, respiration and the control of body temperature (**homeostasis**), are controlled by the brain.

Damage to the brain, when severe enough and when affecting the areas responsible for these basic functions, will result in death.

Information required by the brain to maintain these functions is received from the body and its surroundings by certain types of nerves, and the necessary adjustments required to allow the body to respond to this information is then transmitted from the brain to the body by other types of nerves.

TYPES OF NERVES

Explained in simple terms, the peripheral nervous system is composed of various types of nerves, each with their own specific functions. The cells of the brain receive information from the body and its surroundings via one type of nerve, and they analyse and interpret this information in various areas of the brain itself.

Once interpreted, the brain sends messages to the relevant parts of the body to act on the information accordingly, via various other types of nerves.

Basic Guide to Anatomy and Physiology for Dental Care Professionals, First Edition. Carole Hollins.
© 2012 John Wiley & Sons, Ltd. Published 2012 by John Wiley & Sons, Ltd.

Sensory nerves – carry information from the body to the brain, to be interpreted and acted upon. The information they carry includes the following sensations:

- Pain
- Temperature – both hot and cold
- Touch
- Specialised sensations – sight, sound, taste, smell

Motor nerves – carry information from the brain to the body, to allow the body to respond to the information received accordingly.

The motor nerves can be sub-divided further, depending on their function:

- **Somatic nerves** – carrying impulses to the **musculoskeletal system,** to allow voluntary movement of the body
- **Autonomic nerves** – carrying impulses to blood vessels and internal organs, to effect involuntary actions, such as blood vessel constriction or dilatation:
  - **Sympathetic division** – acts to prepare the body for activity
  - **Parasympathetic division** – acts to restore the body to its 'routine' status
- **Enteric nerves** – carrying impulses specifically to the gastrointestinal tract, to effect peristalsis and digestive secretions, and to regulate blood flow to the area during digestion

Throughout the body, the peripheral nerves travel together, and with blood vessels, in what are known as **neurovascular bundles.**

THE BRAIN AND SPINAL CORD – GROSS ANATOMY

The brain and spinal cord are encased respectively within the skull and the vertebral column of the spine. They are both covered by three membranous layers called the **meninges,** the inner two layers being separated by the **cerebrospinal fluid (CSF).**

This clear fluid is secreted by specialised areas within the brain itself, and it acts in a shock-absorber capacity to protect the brain and spinal cord.

During normal head movements, they both float gently in the CSF and are therefore prevented from 'bouncing around' and becoming damaged within the confines of the skull and vertebral column.

The CSF is formed in a structure called the **choroid plexus,** and it flows from within the deeper structure of the brain out to the meningeal spaces. Once here, it gradually passes back into the venous blood supply so that fresh CSF is always being stimulated to be produced.

The brain consists mainly of two **cerebral hemispheres,** which take up the vast majority of the skull, and these are formed from four lobes in each hemisphere, named as follows, and in line with the bony plates of the skull itself:

- **Frontal lobes** – forming the forehead region
- **Parietal lobes** – forming the top sides of the head
- **Temporal lobes** – forming the lower sides of the head in the ear region
- **Occipital lobes** – forming the back of the head

The cerebral hemispheres appear as vastly convoluted folds of nerve tissue, the layout of which provides a huge surface area of specialised nerve cells appearing as the characteristic 'grey matter' of the brain itself.

The two cerebral hemispheres are joined centrally by the **corpus callosum**, where nerve fibres from one side of the brain can cross to the other side. Immediately beneath this juncture are the important structures of the mid-brain region:

- **Thalamus** – involved with interpreting information from the sense organs
- **Hypothalamus** – involved with the regulation of the endocrine system (composed of various glands that produce **hormones**)
- **Pituitary gland** – master endocrine gland that controls the activities of other glands within the endocrine system

Beneath the mid-brain region lies the brainstem, composed of the **pons** and the **medulla oblongata**, which merges with the spinal cord.

Behind the mid-brain region, and under the occipital lobes of the cerebrum is the **cerebellum**, or hind-brain. This structure is particularly concerned with balance, posture and the coordination of movement.

The areas of the brain are shown diagrammatically in Figure 5.1.

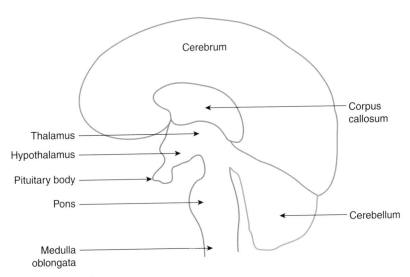

Figure 5.1 Areas of the brain.

NERVOUS SYSTEM

The spinal cord begins as the medulla leaves the skull through the **foramen magnum,** and as the nerve tissue enters the vertebral column. As the cord lies within the bony spine, it gives rise to sequential pairs of nerves along its full length; sensory nerves entering the column and motor nerves leaving it.

These form the **systemic nerves,** which receive sensations from the whole body except the head and neck region, and transmit motor impulses to the same body areas.

The nerves supplying the head and neck region leave the brain directly from its under surface, as 12 pairs of **cranial nerves.**

The cranial nerves

The 12 pairs of cranial nerves are numbered as Roman numerals, but each has its own name too.

Some of the cranial nerves are of particular importance to the dental team because they supply the oral cavity and its surrounding structures. These are covered in detail in several following chapters, and a resume of all 12 is shown in Table 5.1.

Table 5.1 Cranial nerves.

Roman numeral	Name of nerve	Nerve function
I	Olfactory	Sensory – smell
II	Optic	Sensory – sight
III	Occulomotor	Motor – external eye muscles Parasympathetic – pupil size
IV	Trochlear	Motor – external eye muscles
V	**Trigeminal**	**Sensory – pain, temperature, touch of teeth and oral soft tissues** **Motor – muscles of mastication**
VI	Abducens	Motor – external eye muscles
VII	**Facial**	**Sensory – taste from anterior two-third of tongue** **Motor – muscles of facial expression** **Parasympathetic – salivary glands**
VIII	Auditory	Sensory – hearing and balance
IX	**Glossopharyngeal**	**Sensory – taste from posterior tongue** **Motor – control of swallowing** **Parasympathetic – salivary glands**
X	Vagus	Sensory – from the abdominal region Parasympathetic – to the thorax and abdomen
XI	Accessory	Motor – neck muscles and the larynx
XII	**Hypoglossal**	**Motor – tongue muscles**

NERVOUS SYSTEM

Those of particular relevance to the dental team are highlighted in bold.

THE BRAIN – MICROSCOPIC ANATOMY

The tissues of the cerebral hemispheres consist mainly of millions of nerve cells, or **neurones**, with the spaces between filled with supporting cells called **neuroglia**. The whole brain and the spinal cord are bathed in CSF, so that there is no direct contact of the nerve tissue with blood.

The cell bodies of the neurones lie within the outer layer of the brain forming the grey matter of the cortex, while their single thread-like cell extension, or **axon**, all lie within the inner area of the brain, known as the white matter.

Each neurone also has many fine branches extending from the cell body, called **dendrites**, and these lie in close proximity to each other within the grey matter, so that information (as nerve impulses) is rapidly passed from cell to cell.

Once the information received has been analysed and interpreted by the neurones, they send the resultant action information to their target cells along the axon.

The axon itself branches repeatedly as it passes through the body tissues, and each branch ends as a small swelling, called a **nerve terminal**, as it contacts its target cell.

The actual point of contact between the nerve terminal and the target cell is the **synapse**, but microscopically there is no actual contact between the two. Rather, when the nerve impulse arrives at the synapse it causes the release of certain types of chemicals called **neurotransmitters**, and it is these chemicals that continue the electrical transmission to the target cell.

Many successful drugs used in medicine act by preventing the release of the neurotransmitters at the synapse, or by blocking their attachment to the target cells, so that the nerve impulse cannot be transmitted.

A typical neurone is illustrated in Figure 5.2.

As previously described, the target cells are numerous depending on the nerve-generated response required, and may be any of the following examples:

- Skeletal muscle cells, to effect movement
- Specialised muscle cells, such as cardiac muscle, to regulate the heart rate
- Smooth muscle cells, such as in the digestive tract, to effect peristalsis
- Blood vessels, to cause their constriction or dilatation
- Internal organs, to effect cell and/or glandular secretions
- Endocrine glands, to effect or reduce their secretions

The support cells of the brain (and spinal cord) are one of three types, each with their own specific function, as follows:

- **Astrocytes** – star-shaped cells that have direct contact with the outer walls of small blood vessels within the central nervous system (CNS) tissue, forming

NERVOUS SYSTEM

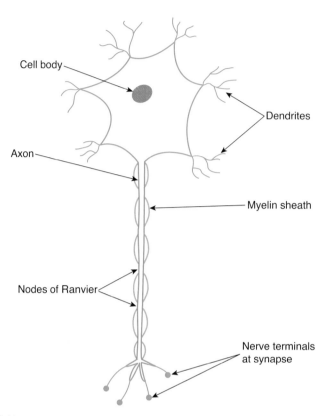

Cell body

Dendrites

Axon

Myelin sheath

Nodes of Ranvier

Nerve terminals
at synapse

Figure 5.2 Neurone.

the **blood–brain barrier;** this prevents the metabolic changes carried by the blood from affecting the normal functioning of the neurones

- **Oligodendrocytes** – form the sectional fatty-tissue sheaths that surround the axon processes of the neurones – the **myelin sheaths.** In the peripheral nervous system, these cells are called **Schwann cells**
- **Microglia** – act as phagocytes within the CNS, congregating wherever injury or infection occurs

The support cells are illustrated in Figure 5.3.

INFORMATION TRANSMISSION BY NERVES

The nervous system is probably the most complicated of all the body systems with regard to the many functions it performs, and its importance in relation to the survival of the organism. However, the way in which it carries out its functions could not be simpler.

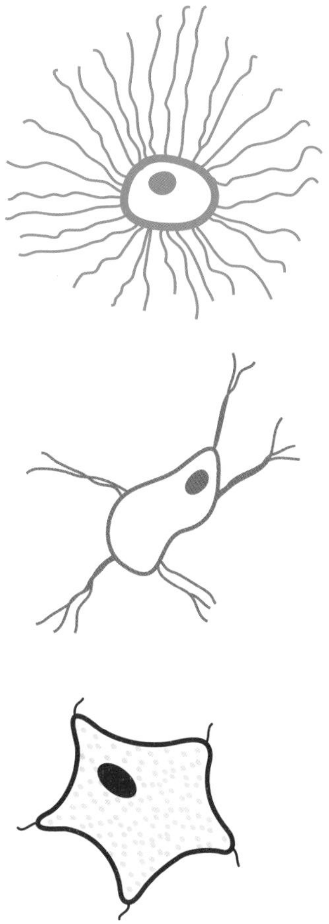

Astrocyte – star-shaped with many
long dendritic processes

Oligodendrocyte – larger body and
many branching dendritic processes

Microglia – phagocyte with few
dendritic processes

Figure 5.3 Support cells of the brain.

All information that passes from the body and the external environment to the brain, its analysis, interpretation and the actions that are generated as a consequence, is transmitted as **simple electrical impulses** throughout the nervous system.

At rest, the nerve cell axons have more of the element **potassium** inside them (as ions), while the outside of the axon has a greater concentration of **sodium ions** in the surrounding fluid of the nerve cell.

This difference in chemical ions is common to all body cells, and the movement of these ions (along with other chemicals and molecules, such as oxygen or glucose) is seen time and again when studying biology and physiology, and explaining how the body works.

Both potassium ions and sodium ions have a positive electrical charge, and while the potassium ions can passively move out of the axons by diffusion, sodium ions cannot move passively in the opposite direction.

With time then, there is a gradual build-up of **negative electrical charge** within the axon as more positive ions move out, and an associated increase in the **positive electrical charge** in the surrounding extracellular fluid.

This potential difference in electrical charge across the axon membrane is called the **membrane potential**.

The potassium ions do not just diffuse out of the axon indiscriminately, but move across the membrane through specific **ion channels** along a concentration gradient. These ion channels can be actively opened by cells to allow controlled ion movement across their membranes under two circumstances:

- In the presence of certain specific chemical agents (such as hormones, drugs, etc.)
- When the membrane potential alters, due to a wave of electrical activity

In the case of axons, the wave of electrical activity is called the **nerve impulse**. When stimulated electrically as the nerve impulse travels along the axon, the membrane potential alters as ion channels open and sodium actively moves into the axon and temporarily alters its electrical status – this is called **depolarisation**.

With myelinated axons, the nerve impulse is able to jump across each section of myelin so that depolarisation occurs in a leap-frog style along the axon.

This allows much faster electrical transmission of the nerve impulse, rather than it having to pass along the full length of the nerve from start to finish.

Nerve impulses are therefore able to travel from anywhere in the body to the CNS in fractions of milliseconds.

As the nerve impulse passes, the unstable depolarised condition alters and the ion channels close to sodium at the same time as the potassium ions begin to diffuse out again. The end result is the **repolarisation** of the axon, and the return of the more stable membrane potential.

Incredibly, these simple nerve impulses result in a multitude of events; ranging from simple muscle contractions, through glandular secretions and normal bodily functions, to such complicated processes as sight, taste, thought and memory.

The electrical transmission event is illustrated in Figure 5.4.

Action of local anaesthetics on nerves

Local anaesthetics are used throughout dentistry to allow the dental team to carry out uncomfortable dental procedures on patients painlessly.

Their method of action is quite simple – they prevent the conduction of the nerve impulse along the axon by preventing the sodium ion channels from opening, and thereby preventing the occurrence of depolarisation.

Local anaesthetics can be applied directly to the oral mucous membranes, as a **topical anaesthetic** that acts directly to anaesthetise that area alone – these

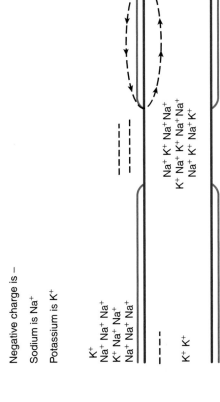

Figure 5.4 Electrical transmission mechanism.

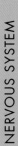

are generally used at the site of an oral injection, to make the needle piercing a less uncomfortable procedure.

Alternatively, when a more profound action is required, the local anaesthetic can be injected through the oral membrane into a localised region around the nerves to be anaesthetised. The two basic techniques are as follows:

- **Infiltration injection** – the needle tip is inserted just below the surface of the mucous membrane, and the solution released there so that it can be absorbed by superficial nerves directly
- **Nerve block injection** – the needle tip is carefully positioned deep in the oral tissues, within millimetres of a main nerve trunk (such as the inferior dental nerve), and the solution released there to block the whole nerve trunk

Dental local anaesthetics can also be given into the periodontal ligament of a tooth (**intraligamentary injection**), or through the alveolar bone so that the solution is deposited close to the roots of the teeth (**intra-osseous injection**).

Many modern local anaesthetics also contain chemicals that act to cause blood vessel contraction in the area of use, thereby extending the time period of anaesthesia.

These chemicals are called **vasoconstrictors** and the most frequently used in dentistry are adrenaline and felypressin.

NERVOUS SYSTEM MEDICAL CONDITIONS

Stroke (cerebrovascular accident)

The blood supply to the brain is well controlled by numerous normal body mechanisms – indeed, at times of severe blood loss or reduced blood oxygenation, the body will selectively divert blood from other organs to the brain, in an attempt to maintain the cerebral circulation.

A stroke occurs when there is a sudden alteration in cerebral blood flow, due to one of three events:

- **Cerebral thrombosis** – the formation of a blood clot within a brain artery, reducing or cutting off the oxygenated blood supply to that region (in a similar fashion to the onset of a heart attack when a coronary artery is blocked)
- **Cerebral embolism** – the blockage of a brain artery by a loose blood clot formed elsewhere in the body, that detaches from the blood vessel wall and circulates to the brain
- **Cerebral haemorrhage** – when a cerebral blood vessel ruptures and bleeding occurs within the skull, causing increasing pressure on the brain

The effects of a severe stroke are of sudden onset, but will depend on the area of the brain affected as to the signs that will occur.

As the axons of the nerve cells on each side of the brain cross-over in the corpus callosum, the signs shown by the stroke victim will affect the opposite side – so a left-sided stroke will cause right-sided musculoskeletal signs of weakness or even paralysis. In addition, speech is affected when a left-sided stroke occurs.

Strokes due to cerebral haemorrhage will be treated by the successful management of the haemorrhage itself.

Transient ischaemic attack

When a small, partial blockage of a cerebral artery occurs, the signs and symptoms are far less dramatic – often exhibiting just as a mild visual disturbance or a brief memory lapse lasting minutes. This is known as a transient ischaemic attack, or TIA.

The sufferer will make a full recovery, but the experience is actually a warning signal that a full-blown stroke could occur in future, in a similar way to angina attacks having the potential to develop into a full myocardial infarction. The TIA indicates that part of the brain has a reduced blood flow.

Bell's palsy

A (usually) temporary paralysis of the VII cranial nerve – the facial nerve.

It often occurs following any condition causing inflammation in the region of the facial nerve, and results in a one-sided weakness of the facial muscles.

In particular, any inflammation associated with the parotid salivary glands can result in Bell's palsy, as the facial nerve runs across and through this gland to reach the oral cavity. It does not supply the gland itself though.

The condition of Bell's palsy is self-limiting, and subsides as the inflammation resolves.

Epilepsy

When the usually well-organised and regulated electrical activity of the nerve cells in the brain becomes temporarily abnormal and disorganised, the sufferer is said to have a **seizure**. During a seizure, the normal electrical discharges of the nerve cells become completely chaotic and random, and are often started by a stimulus such as flashing lights.

Sufferers experiencing a tendency to seizures are diagnosed as having epilepsy.

The two main types of generalised seizure, where consciousness is lost, are:

- **Grand mal seizure** – the sufferer falls down unconscious, the body stiffens and becomes rigid and then twitches and jerks uncontrollably – these signs are referred to as **tonic–clonic seizures**

- **Petit mal seizure** – the sufferer has only a momentary loss of consciousness, with no associated abnormal movements, indeed they often are thought to be just daydreaming for a period of just seconds – their alternative name is therefore **absence seizures**

While petit mal seizures last just seconds, grand mal seizures can last up to 5 minutes before the tonic–clonic phase ends and consciousness returns. In both cases, the sufferer has no memory of the seizure and especially after a grand mal event, is often confused and disorientated for a time.

When a grand mal seizure lasts for more than 5 minutes, or repeat seizures occur rapidly after the first, the sufferer is said to be in **status epilepticus** – an often fatal condition requiring urgent emergency medical treatment.

Meningitis

This condition occurs due to inflammation of the meninges, the membranous layers that cover the brain and spinal cord.

The inflammation occurs due to infection of the meninges by either a virus or a bacterium, the latter being the far more serious of the two.

The infective organism usually arrives at the meninges via the blood from an infection elsewhere in the body, although it can occur initially as an ear or sinus infection and pass directly to the skull chamber.

Viral meningitis commonly occurs during the winter months, is usually not serious and requires no treatment for the sufferer to recover.

Bacterial meningitis, especially **meningococcal meningitis**, is far more serious and even life-threatening if not diagnosed and treated promptly, due to the raised intracranial pressure produced by the inflammation, which causes damage to the brain itself.

NERVOUS SYSTEM MEDICATIONS

Stroke

The aim of drug therapy is to destroy any blood clots, limit the damage caused by the blockage to the cerebral circulation and prevent the recurrence of clot formation:

- **Clot busters** – various **thrombolytic** drugs that act to encourage the destruction of the clot tissue itself
- **Anticoagulants** – to prevent further thrombus formation, especially as a deep vein thrombosis, initially as fast-acting **heparin**, and then as long-term **warfarin**
- **Aspirin** – to prevent further clot formation by preventing platelet aggregation

Transient ischaemic attack

The aim of drug therapy is to prevent further attacks, by reducing the chances of further clot formation:

- **Aspirin** – given as a daily dose (usually 75 mg) to prevent platelet aggregation and reduce the chances of embolus formation
- **Warfarin** – which acts by inhibiting the formation of various clotting factors in the liver, so that the clotting cascade cannot occur effectively

Sufferers on long-term aspirin therapy will have 'thin blood' and may bleed profusely after dental extractions. This can be avoided by temporarily stopping the medication prior to the extraction, and by careful post-operative management of haemostasis using sutures and haemostatic sponges.

Warfarin may also cause abnormal, and more profound, bleeding in users, so their clotting time is carefully controlled by dose regulation.

Users undergo regular blood tests to determine their **INR levels** (international normalised ratio), which should be kept between 2 and 4, by warfarin dose manipulation.

If higher than 4, patients should be referred to hospital for dental extractions, where bleeding can be carefully monitored and controlled. If lower than 2, there is a risk of clot formation.

Epilepsy

The aim of drug therapy is to reduce the risk of a seizure occurring:

- **Anticonvulsants** – especially **phenytoin** and **carbamazepine,** which are taken for life and prevent the occurrence of aberrant electrical discharges in the brain

Phenytoin has several side effects, including the onset of gingival hyperplasia.

Patients may have to undergo repeated gingivectomy procedures when gingival overgrowth prevents adequate routine oral hygiene levels from being maintained.

The gingival hyperplasia is exacerbated, but not caused by, the presence of dental plaque.

Meningitis

Bacterial meningitis is a life-threatening condition, which requires hospitalisation and urgent treatment with intravenous antibiotics to avoid permanent brain damage or death.

NERVOUS SYSTEM

Chapter 6
Oral embryology and histology

DEFINITIONS

Oral embryology is the study of the development of the oral cavity, and the structures within it, during the formation and development of the embryo in the first 8 weeks of pregnancy.

After this point, the unborn child is referred to as a foetus.

The correct biological term for this time period before birth is **prenatal**.

Histology is the specialised biological area of study concerned with the microscopic structure and function of tissues.

This chapter will cover the embryological development of all oral structures, as well as the basic histology of the embryonic tissues.

The histology of the following dentally relevant structures warrant more detailed notes, and are discussed elsewhere:

- Tooth histology – covered in Chapter 8
- Periodontal histology – covered in Chapter 9
- Salivary gland histology – covered in Chapter 10

OVERVIEW OF GENERAL EMBRYO DEVELOPMENT

To understand the embryological development of the oral tissues, the dental care professional (DCP) needs to have a basic knowledge of the process of embryo formation, and the significance of the origins of various body tissues and organs to help understand how congenital defects, pathology and disease processes occur.

The 8-week time span of the embryo is summarised in the following text.

Following fertilisation of the female egg by male sperm, the resultant single cell, or **zygote**, travels to the womb (uterus) while undergoing repeated cell

---

Basic Guide to Anatomy and Physiology for Dental Care Professionals, First Edition. Carole Hollins.
© 2012 John Wiley & Sons, Ltd. Published 2012 by John Wiley & Sons, Ltd.

divisions that double the number of cells present; from one to two, then to four, then eight, and so on.

At about 6 days after fertilisation, the cluster of cells so produced then forms into two distinct groups, with the outer layer of cells forming a wall around the inner group, and they develop as follows:

- Outer wall – attaches the cell group into the lining of the uterus, and forms the **placenta**
- Inner cluster – expands to form the **embryo**

The inner cells then organise themselves into a flat disc, eventually containing three distinct layers of cells (and one sub-layer) from which all the tissues and organs will develop:

- **Ectoderm layer** – outer layer of cells, which form the outer skin layer, the sensory cells of the eyes, ears and nose, some of the nervous system and external skin glands
- **Neuroectoderm cells** – specialised cells from the ectoderm layer, and which form connective tissue, cartilage, some bone and some dental tissues
- **Mesoderm layer** – middle layer of cells, which form the deep skin layer, muscle, bone marrow and blood cells, lymphatic system, reproductive organs and excretory organs including the salivary glands
- **Endoderm layer** – inner layer of cells, which form the linings of the respiratory and digestive systems, liver and pancreas

The space between this disc and the outer wall of cells develops as the amniotic sac.

The development of the embryo from weeks 3 to 8 is then rapid and astounding, and is summarised in the following text.

Third week – see Figure 6.1

- Disc of cells becomes pear shaped and develops a head end and a tail end
- Rod of cells develops along the back of the embryo to form the **notochord**, which develops into the spine
- Embryo now has two symmetrical halves – left and right
- Notochord rolls to form a tubular structure that later develops into the brain and spinal cord

Fourth week – see Figure 6.2

- Cells along the back of the embryo grow more rapidly than the front, forming a curved shape
- Endoderm tissue buds begin developing, and will later form the respiratory and digestive organs

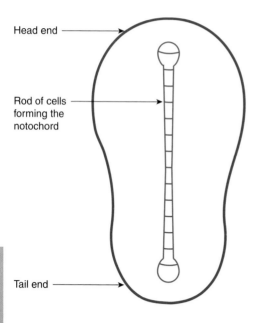

Head end

Rod of cells forming the notochord

Tail end

Figure 6.1 Third-week embryo.

- Brain begins to develop, as do eye stalks and ear pits
- Ectoderm tissue buds develop, and will later form the limbs
- Ectoderm tissue folds develop as **branchial arches**, which will become the jaws and other neck structures (in lower life forms such as fish, these structures develop as gills)

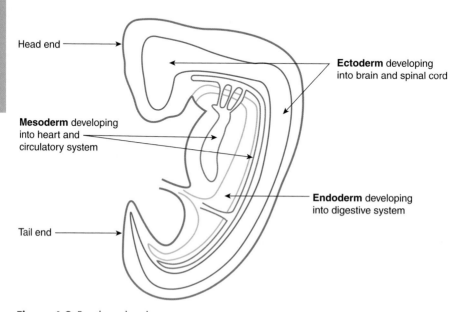

Head end

Ectoderm developing into brain and spinal cord

Mesoderm developing into heart and circulatory system

Endoderm developing into digestive system

Tail end

Figure 6.2 Fourth-week embryo.

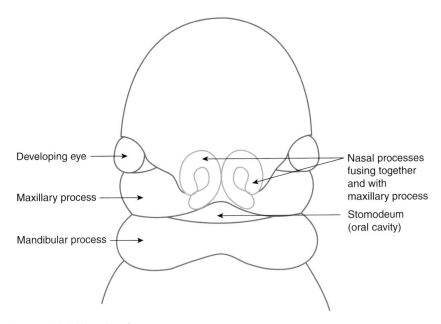

Figure 6.3 Fifth-week embryo.

- Heart begins developing on the front of the embryo, beneath the head, and is pushed down into the chest as the branchial arches develop

Fifth week – see Figure 6.3

- Nose begins developing as nasal pits
- Jaws and ears form
- Hands and feet begin developing
- All internal organs are developing
- Ectoderm tissue folds grow to join at the front and form the chest and abdominal cavity walls

Sixth week – see Figure 6.4

- Eyes and ears are formed
- Mouth and nose begin to develop

Eighth week – see Figure 6.5

- Face is recognisable
- Embryo curvature relaxes
- Limbs become jointed
- Most internal organs are formed

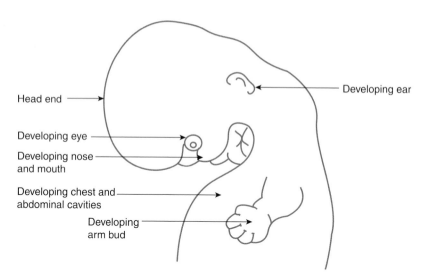

Head end

Developing eye

Developing nose and mouth

Developing chest and abdominal cavities

Developing arm bud

Developing ear

Figure 6.4 Sixth-week embryo.

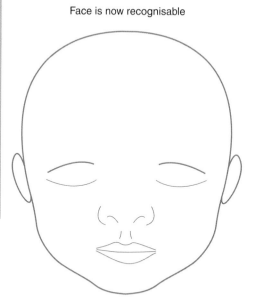

Face is now recognisable

Figure 6.5 Eighth-week embryo.

ORAL EMBRYOLOGY – OVERVIEW

As summarised previously, the majority of oral embryological development occurs between weeks 3 and 8 after conception, and the oral and facial structures are fully formed by week 12.

As the roof of the mouth, the **palate,** forms the floor of the nasal cavity, the development of these two cavities is inextricably linked and will be discussed together.

Third week

- Shallow indentation of the ectoderm at the head end of the embryo develops – this is the primitive mouth, or **stomodeum**
- This is separated from the rudimentary pharynx by a temporary structure called the **oropharyngeal membrane**

Fourth week onwards

- Ectoderm tissue, with considerable neuroectoderm cells present, folds and develops into the six **branchial arches**, which form various oral and neck structures (see Table 6.1)
- Oropharyngeal membrane disintegrates so that the stomodeum becomes deeper and gradually forms the oral cavity
- Two buds of tissue containing cells of all three embryonic layers begin to swell beneath the stomodeum and form the **mandibular processes**
- Once fused together at the front of the embryo, they form the **mandible** and its associated structures
- At the same time, two other tissue buds develop from the mandibular processes, and swell above them to form the back section of the **maxilla** and its associated structures, up to the future position of the canine teeth

Table 6.1 Branchial arches and associated derivative structures.

Arches	Tissues	Nerves and muscles	Bones
First (mandibular)	Teeth, middle and lower face, lips, cheeks and body of tongue	Trigeminal nerve, muscles of mastication and some suprahyoid muscles	Mandible, back part of maxilla, secondary palate, zygomatic bones and some bones of middle ear
Second (hyoid)	Back part of tongue, various ligaments between skull and mandible	Facial nerve, muscles of facial expression and some suprahyoid muscles	Middle ear bone, part of temporal bone and part of hyoid bone
Third	Back part of tongue	Glossopharyngeal nerve and some pharyngeal muscles	Part of hyoid bone
Fourth to sixth	Back part of tongue	Muscles of larynx and pharynx and vagus nerve	Laryngeal cartilages

ORAL EMBRYOLOGY AND HISTOLOGY

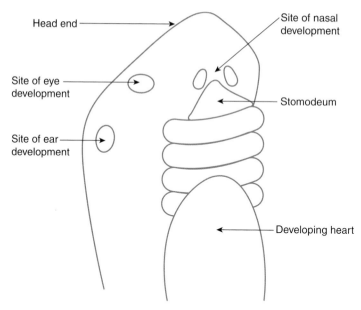

Figure 6.6 Early facial development.

- Above the stomodeum, yet another tissue bud develops and forms the **frontonasal process**
- This goes on to develop the upper face, the nasal structures and the front section of the palate at the future position of the incisor teeth (see Figure 6.6)

- The front section of the palate is called the **primary palate**, while the back section is the **secondary palate**
- The primary palate develops in one piece, while the secondary palate develops as two shelves that join at the midline from week 6 (see Figure 6.7)

An understanding of the embryological development of the face and oral cavity helps to explain the cranial nerve supply of the head and neck region, which can otherwise seem a disconcerting area of study to some DCPs.

Embryological development of the tongue

By the fourth week of embryological development, the primitive pharynx has been formed by the first four branchial arches. It is present at this stage as the top end of the hollow tube that will go on to develop into the respiratory and digestive systems. The seal of the oropharyngeal membrane has disintegrated, and the stomodeum is deepening to form the oral cavity.

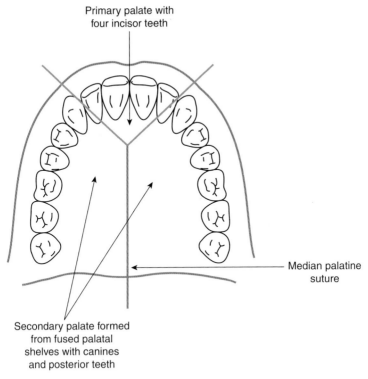

Primary palate with
four incisor teeth

Median palatine
suture

Secondary palate formed
from fused palatal
shelves with canines
and posterior teeth

Figure 6.7 The palate.

At this point, tissue buds develop on the floor of the primitive pharynx; those from the first branchial arches develop into the body of the tongue, while those from the second, third and fourth branchial arches eventually develop into the base of the tongue:

- A central tissue bud called the **tuberculum impar** develops from the first branchial arch
- Two side buds develop next to it as **lateral lingual swellings**
- These two swellings grow together and encompass the first tissue bud, and the resultant organ becomes the body of the tongue, forming the anterior two-thirds of its whole structure
- As the cells along the sides of the lingual swellings disintegrate, the body of the tongue becomes free from the floor of the mouth except for a central tag of tissue beneath, which is the **lingual frenum**
- From the third and fourth branchial arches, another pair of swellings develop, called the **copula,** and these form the base of the tongue
- As the copula grow forwards and encompass tissue from the second branchial arch, they merge with the anterior swellings at around week 8

- The point at which they join is visible as a V-shaped groove called the **sulcus terminalis**
- The inner muscles of the tongue structure are derived from other tissue besides the branchial arches, and are supplied by the hypoglossal nerve
- The various taste buds found on the tongue develop from the eighth week of embryological development, and are discussed further in Chapter 7

Embryological development of the teeth

The primary dentition begins development at about the sixth week of embryological development, and continues in the foetus. The secondary dentition begins development in the foetus, but continues for many years after birth.

Tooth development, or **odontogenesis**, occurs in several stages common to both dentitions. It always begins in the anterior mandibular region, then the anterior maxillary region and then progresses posteriorly in both arches as the jaws grow in length.

At the sixth week of embryological development, the stomodeum is lined by ectoderm, which forms the oral epithelium and has a layer of neuroectoderm cells beneath. These two cell layers are separated by a **basement membrane**.

Odontogenesis occurs in four distinct stages, as described in the following text, and as shown in Figure 6.8.

Initiation stage – weeks 6–7
- Oral epithelium grows down into the deeper tissues, producing a layer called the **dental lamina**
- This growth occurs at ten distinct points along each future jaw, to eventually form the 20 teeth of the primary dentition
- Growth begins in the lower anterior area, then the upper anterior area and then progresses posteriorly in both arches

Bud stage – week 8
- Dental lamina continues to grow into the deeper tissues of the jaws, to form a bud shape at each growth point
- Dental lamina and jaw are still separated by the basement membrane
- There is no differentiation of the tissues into anything resembling a tooth at this stage

Cap stage – weeks 9–10
- Dental lamina continues to grow, but does so unevenly so that a cap shape is produced
- Cell differentiation now occurs to form three distinct areas within the tooth bud structure, which is now called a **tooth germ**
- Outer, cap-shaped layer now called the **enamel organ**, which develops into **enamel**

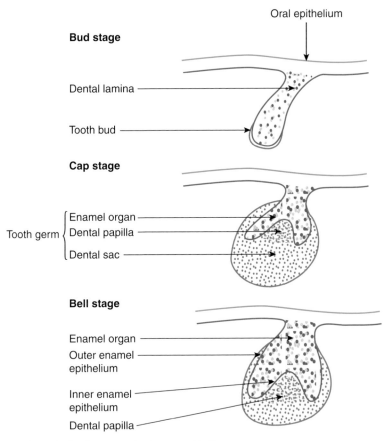

Figure 6.8 Tooth development – bud, cap and bell stages.

- Inner condensed tissue surrounded by the cap structure, referred to as the **dental papilla,** which develops into both **dentine** and **pulp**
- Surrounding condensed mass of tissue, called the **dental sac,** which develops into the supporting structures of the tooth – **cementum, periodontal ligament** and **alveolar bone**

Bell stage – weeks 11–12
- Further cell differentiation occurs in all three areas of the tooth germ
- Enamel organ continues growing and appears bell shaped
- Several cell layers develop, the outer ones as protective layers for the enamel organ and the innermost layer develops into **ameloblasts,** the cells that lay down enamel
- Basement membrane gradually disappears, but continues to separate the enamel organ from the dental papilla, and is referred to as the **amelodentinal junction**

- Outer layer of cells in the dental papilla develop into **odontoblasts,** which lay down dentine
- Inner layer of cells develop into the dental pulp tissue
- Dental sac tissue gradually differentiates past this point into connective tissue and bone, eventually forming the supporting structures of the tooth

Once the crown of the tooth has developed, the cells lying at the very lowest tips of the enamel organ, including the future ameloblasts, organise themselves into a structure known as the **cervical loop.**

They grow deep into the dental sac tissue and enclose dental papilla tissue as they do so. The resulting elongated structure is called **Hertwig's root sheath,** and the dental papilla tissue it encloses gradually forms the dentine and pulp structure of the tooth root.

In multi-rooted teeth (molars and upper first premolars), the root sheath splits to develop the correct number of roots per tooth.

Apposition and maturation

Once the crown and root areas of the tooth germs are formed, the final stages of the process involve the sequential layering formation of enamel, dentine and cementum, and then their calcification.

These stages are referred to as **apposition** and **maturation,** respectively.

DEVELOPMENTAL DISTURBANCES AFFECTING LIP AND PALATE

Cleft lip

This condition occurs when one or both of the maxillary processes fail to fuse with the nasal process in the embryo, resulting in either a unilateral (one-sided) or bilateral (both sides) cleft lip.

Depending on the severity of the deformity produced, treatment is via oral and plastic surgery initially, and may involve aesthetic dental treatment and speech therapy.

Cleft palate

As shown in Figure 6.7, the hard and soft palates develop from three sections – the primary palate and the two shelves of the secondary palate.

Failure of any of these sections to join and fuse together during embryological development will result in a cleft palate, and the severity of the defect produced depends on where the failure occurs.

Failure of the shelves of the secondary palate to fuse together results in the oral and nasal cavities being open to each other, to a greater or lesser degree.

Failure of one or both sides of the primary palate to fuse with the secondary palate can occur, and often involves a unilateral or bilateral cleft lip too.

Failure of all three sections of the palate to fuse together results in the most serious defect of all, but all clefts are amenable to corrective oral and plastic surgery, with dental intervention and speech therapy as necessary.

Corrective surgery is usually begun within 3 months of birth, especially if the baby experiences difficulty with suckling and feeding.

DEVELOPMENTAL DISTURBANCES AFFECTING TEETH

Initiation stage

If the process of initiation does not occur, then one or several teeth will not form. This is only of consequence when the secondary dentition is involved, and the teeth usually affected are as follows, in order of frequency:

- Upper lateral incisors
- One or more of the third molars
- Lower second premolars

The term **anodontia** describes the absence of all teeth, while the term **partial anodontia** describes the absence of some teeth.

The condition may arise due to infection, radiation exposure, metabolic dysfunction, genetics or due to syndromes affecting the development of tissues of ectodermal origin, as in **ectodermal dysplasia**.

On the other hand, if the initiation stage occurs profusely, one or more 'extra' teeth will develop. These are referred to as **supernumerary teeth**, are usually smaller than normal teeth and conical in shape, and tend to be an incidental finding on routine dental radiographs.

In order of frequency, their positions are as follows:

- Between the upper central incisors, and specifically called **mesiodens** when present here
- Behind the upper third molars
- In the premolar region of both arches

Depending on their position, they may cause localised crowding or prevent the eruption of the secondary dentition, and are then best extracted.

Bud stage

Excessive proliferation of the dental lamina tissues at this stage will result in abnormally large teeth, and the condition is referred to as **macrodontia**.

ORAL EMBRYOLOGY AND HISTOLOGY

Conversely, a reduction in proliferation will result in abnormally small teeth, which is a condition referred to as **microdontia**.

Hereditary factors are commonly involved in either proliferation abnormality, and the teeth usually affected are:

- Upper permanent lateral incisors, and referred to as **peg laterals**
- Third molars

Cap stage

Any disturbance of the development of the various tissues at this stage, or of their cell differentiation, will result in one of several anomalies.

Dens in dente

When the enamel organ grows abnormally and pushes further into the dental papilla than is usual, the resulting tooth is referred to as **dens in dente** (appears as a 'tooth within a tooth' radiographically).

This condition most frequently affects the upper permanent incisors, especially the lateral incisors. The affected tooth has a deep pit palatally, which may compromise the pulp itself and result in an exposure, requiring endodontic treatment to save the tooth from extraction.

Gemination

If the tooth germ attempts to divide in two during the cap stage, the resultant single tooth has an enlarged pulp chamber and the crown appears as an enlarged and 'twinned' structure. This is caused by **gemination**, and can occur in both the primary and secondary dentition. It usually affects anterior teeth, and may therefore have aesthetic implications as the affected tooth can appear abnormally enlarged.

Fusion

Conversely, when two adjacent tooth germs join together at the cap stage, it is referred to as **fusion**. Radiographically, the abnormally large crown of the tooth will exhibit two pulp chambers, although it usually has just one root. This condition usually affects anterior teeth of the primary dentition.

Tubercles

These are additional cusp-like structures on the crown of the tooth, most often affecting the permanent molars, especially the third molars.

ORAL EMBRYOLOGY AND HISTOLOGY

They may also occur palatally as extensions in the cingulum area of upper anterior teeth.

Apposition and maturation stages
Any factor that disturbs the laying down and/or calcification of enamel or dentine results in a group of conditions called **dysplasias**.

Enamel dysplasia
These may occur due to local factors, such as trauma or infection, or systemic factors, such as excessive intake of fluoride.

Local factors affect one or a few teeth only, appearing as pitting or grooving of the enamel surface.

Systemic factors affect all teeth undergoing enamel calcification at the time, resulting in widespread pitting and grooving, as appears with **enamel fluorosis**.

When the dysplasia has a hereditary origin, all teeth are affected, and one particular example is **amelogenesis imperfecta**. This literally means the faulty laying down and calcification of the enamel, which is consequently thin and breaks off the tooth structure easily.

The underlying exposed dentine gives the teeth an unsightly yellow appearance, and the crowns are easily worn down during normal masticatory use, by attrition.

Extensive restorative dental treatment is usually required to protect the teeth from attrition, and improve the aesthetics.

Dentine dysplasia
This occurs less frequently than enamel dysplasia, and the only condition of note is of a hereditary origin and is called **dentinogenesis imperfecta**.

The affected teeth have an unusual grey or brown appearance, and although the enamel is normal it breaks off easily due to lack of support from the underlying faulty dentine.

Again, extensive restorative dental treatment is required.

Tooth Eruption
Both the primary and secondary dentition usually erupt in a chronological order, by the sequential vertical movement of each tooth into the oral cavity during **active eruption**.

Microscopically, active eruption can be easily described, but the actual reason why teeth erupt is theoretical, and beyond the scope of this text.

Active eruption

Once apposition and maturation of the tooth crown are complete, the eruption events are as follows:

- Tooth crown is covered by a **cuticle** with a reduced epithelial layer between it and the enamel surface
- This reduced epithelial layer is called the **reduced enamel epithelium**, and it fuses with that of the oral cavity
- At the point of fusion, the cells disintegrate to produce a 'tunnel' through which the tooth can then actively erupt
- The associated discomfort of this cell disintegration is known as **teething**
- A circular seal of tissue always remains at the neck of the tooth during eruption, and this later becomes the **junctional epithelium**
- This process is the same for both dentitions

Primary exfoliation and secondary replacement

As active eruption of the permanent dentition begins, the primary teeth need to be lost from the oral cavity to make way for their secondary successors. The process is as follows:

- All secondary teeth except the upper incisors begin developing on the palatal or lingual sides of their primary predecessors
- As they develop, the bone between them is removed by specialised cells called **osteoclasts**
- At the same time, some specialise further and develop into **odontoclast cells**, which remove the primary tooth roots
- This latter process is called **resorption**
- As the primary tooth is eaten away, it gradually loosens and can be pulled out or allowed to exfoliate naturally
- The crown of the permanent tooth usually erupts into the oral cavity at the same time, or just after exfoliation, by the process of active eruption described previously

During tooth development, a failure of the reduced enamel epithelium and the oral cavity epithelium to fuse together will allow the development of an abnormal sac around the tooth. This is known as an **eruption cyst.**

The cyst appears as a bluish soft mass over the bulge of the unerupted tooth, and usually disintegrates as the tooth eventually erupts.

When the cyst occurs over an impacted tooth that cannot erupt naturally, it becomes known as a **dentigerous cyst.** They occur especially around the third molars, and their growth may push adjacent teeth out of line, or even compromise the jawbone. They require full surgical removal, as they can become cancerous if left in place.

ORAL HISTOLOGY – ORAL MUCOSA

The histology of the teeth, the periodontium and the salivary glands are covered in Chapters 8, 9 and 10, respectively.

The whole of the mouth is lined with epithelial mucosal tissue, although the histological structure of it varies regionally throughout the oral cavity.

In general, the oral mucosal epithelium is composed of up to four basic layers:

- **Epithelium** – forming the outer layer, which is the visible surface of the oral mucosa
- **Basement membrane** – separating the epithelium from the next layer
- **Lamina propria** – middle layer composed of tight connective tissue
- **Submucosa** – deepest layer, composed of loose connective tissue with other structures present (such as fat or muscle cells), but this layer does not occur in all regions of the oral cavity

There are three variations in the regional appearance of the oral mucosa, which have therefore been classified as three distinct histological types, as follows:

- Lining mucosa
- Masticatory mucosa
- Specialised mucosa

Lining mucosa

As the name suggests, this lines the oral cavity in the following areas, and provides a physical barrier between anything that enters the mouth and its deeper structures:

- All alveolar, buccal and labial mucosa (so inner surfaces of cheeks and lips)
- Floor of the mouth
- Underside of tongue (known as the ventral surface)
- Soft palate

Its physical appearance is as a smooth, moist surface, which can be stretched and comfortably squashed, so that it can act as a cushioning tissue to the underlying structures.

Microscopically, these functions are achieved by the following histological features:

- Non-keratinised epithelium on the surface
- Smooth basement membrane
- Elastic fibres within the lamina propria, allowing the tissue to stretch
- Presence of submucosa to act as a cushion

ORAL EMBRYOLOGY AND HISTOLOGY

Masticatory mucosa

This regional variation occurs over structures directly involved in masticatory actions (chewing) or with the phonetic formation of sounds during speech:

- Attached gingivae
- Top side of tongue (known as the dorsal surface)
- Hard palate

The mucosa is tight and firmly attached to its underlying structures, and has a hard-wearing surface to prevent traumatic damage when coming in contact with food particles, chemicals, oral hygiene products, and so on.

Microscopically, these functions are achieved by the following histological features:

- Keratinised surface epithelium, providing a tough, protective surface made of the protein, keratin (also covers skin, nails and hair)
- Highly ridged basement membrane, forming a firm base for the tissue and accounting for the stippled appearance of the gingivae and the ridged front area of the hard palate
- This mucosa forms the **mucoperiosteum** of the underlying alveolar bone in the dental arches and in the hard palate
- No elastic fibres present
- No submucosa present

Specialised mucosa

This occurs only on the dorsal and lateral surfaces of the tongue.

These tongue surfaces are covered with normal masticatory mucosa, with the specialised mucosa interspersed as discrete tissue areas called **lingual papillae.**

There are four types of lingual papillae found on the tongue, and three of them contain specialised areas of tissue formed into **taste buds**, which allow the sensation of taste. The four types are:

- **Filiform papillae** – cover the majority of the dorsal tongue surface, giving it a velvety appearance, contain no taste buds and act to help guide food towards the throat for swallowing
- **Fungiform papillae** – less frequent occurrence and appear as red dots over the dorsum of the tongue, contain taste buds that detect sweet, salt and some sour taste sensations
- **Foliate papillae** – lie along the sides of the tongue towards the back, contain taste buds that mainly detect sour and salt taste sensations
- **Circumvallate papillae** – lie just in front of the sulcus terminalis in a corresponding 'V' shape, contain taste buds that detect bitter taste sensations

The usual positioning of the various types of taste bud across the tongue is shown in Figure 6.9.

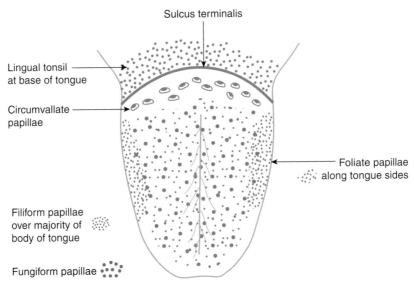

Sulcus terminalis

Lingual tonsil
at base of tongue

Circumvallate
papillae

Foliate papillae
along tongue sides

Filiform papillae
over majority of
body of tongue

Fungiform papillae

Figure 6.9 Tongue with taste bud distribution.

HISTOLOGY OF THE TASTE BUDS AND TASTE SENSATION

Each type of lingual papillae involved with taste sensation appears microscopically as more or less mushroom-shaped structures, with their outer epithelial layer containing the taste buds themselves.

The taste buds are made up of just two cell types – (1) **taste cells** and (2) **supporting cells**, all elongated and arranged in an oblong-shaped structure running from the basement membrane to the surface of the papilla, as shown in Figure 6.10.

The inner core of cells tends to be composed of the taste cells, and these are in contact with the oral cavity at the **taste pore**. Here, the cells have surface taste receptors that are stimulated when they come into contact with dissolved food particles within the oral cavity.

The stimulation produced is transmitted to the base of the taste cells, where sensory nerve endings are located. These in turn transmit the stimulation as an electrical impulse to the brain, where it is processed, analysed and identified as one of the taste sensations – sweet, salt, sour or bitter, or more usually a combination of these sensations.

The cranial nerves involved with the transmission of these sensory nerve impulses are:

- **Facial nerve** – cranial nerve VII, transmitting from the anterior two-thirds of the tongue

ORAL EMBRYOLOGY AND HISTOLOGY

ORAL EMBRYOLOGY AND HISTOLOGY

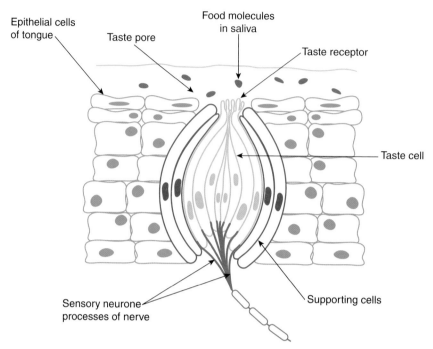

Epithelial cells of tongue

Taste pore

Food molecules in saliva

Taste receptor

Taste cell

Sensory neurone processes of nerve

Supporting cells

Figure 6.10 Taste bud.

- **Glossopharyngeal nerve** – cranial nerve IX, transmitting from the posterior one-third of the tongue

The complicated and coordinated movements of the tongue that occur during speech, mastication and swallowing are controlled by the **hypoglossal nerve** (cranial nerve XII), and are covered in Chapter 7.

Chapter 7
Skull and oral anatomy

SKULL ANATOMY – OVERVIEW

The skull is the topmost part of the bony skeleton of the body, the head, and is made up of two main areas:

- **Cranium** – the hollow cavity that surrounds the brain
- **Face** – the front vertical part of the skull, containing the orbital, nasal and oral cavities and the jaws

All of the bones of the skull except the lower jaw, the **mandible**, are fixed to each other by immovable joints called **sutures**.

The base of the cranium articulates with the topmost bone of the vertebral column, the **atlas**, allowing nodding movements of the head.

At birth and during infancy, the bony plates making up the cranium are separated from each other by two natural membrane covered spaces called **fontanelles**, which allow growth of the brain without bony restriction.

By the age of 18 months the fontanelles should have closed, following the natural growth together of the bony plates making up the cranium.

ANATOMY OF THE CRANIUM

The cranium is composed of eight bones, which are separated by the cranial sutures – these are visible on a dry skull as the zig-zagged joints between the bony plates.

The bones themselves are as follows:

- **Frontal bone** – single plate at the front of the cranium above the eyes, forming the forehead
- **Parietal bones** – pair of plates forming the top and the greater area of the sides of the cranium

Basic Guide to Anatomy and Physiology for Dental Care Professionals, First Edition. Carole Hollins.
© 2012 John Wiley & Sons, Ltd. Published 2012 by John Wiley & Sons, Ltd.

- **Temporal bones** – pair of fan-shaped plates in the temple region of the lower sides of the cranium, in front of the ears
- **Occipital bone** – single plate at the back and partial underside of the cranium
- **Sphenoid bone** – single plate forming the majority of the base of the cranium
- **Ethmoid bone** – single plate at the lower front of the cranium, immediately behind the nose

The skull and cranial bones are illustrated in Figure 7.1.

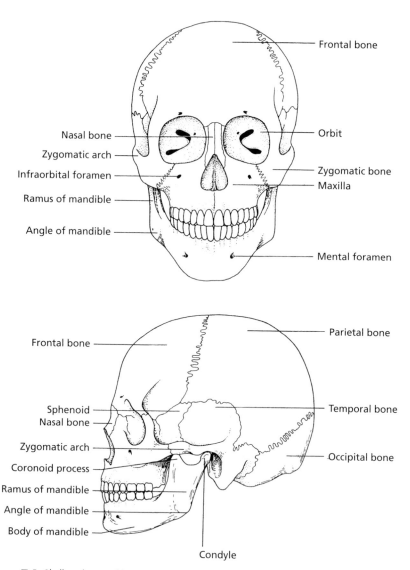

Figure 7.1 Skull and cranial bones. (From Hollins, C. (2008). *Levison's Textbook for Dental Nurses*, 10th edn. Blackwell Publishing, Oxford. Reproduced with permission from John Wiley & Sons, Ltd.)

The main function of the cranium is to encase and protect the brain.

All of the sensory nerve cells running from the body to the brain, and all of the motor nerves running from the brain to the body have to pass in and out of this bony cavity, and they do so through many natural openings in the underside of the cranium, called **foramina** (singular – **foramen**).

Similarly, all of the blood vessels supplying the head and neck structures pass through these same foramina or between natural spaces between adjacent bones, called **fissures**.

The largest foramen of all is the **foramen magnum**, which opens through the occipital bone, and allows the exit of the spinal cord from the base of the brain and into the vertebral column of the spine.

Other foramina of the cranium with particular relevance to dentistry are shown in Table 7.1.

Some of the bony openings are listed and their positions on the underside of the cranium are shown in Figure 7.2.

In addition to these bony openings, some cranial bones also have various projections and plates present on their outer surfaces, which serve as attachments for ligaments and muscles associated with head and jaw movements, or which form part of facial structures.

Those with particular relevance to dentistry are shown in Table 7.2.

Some of the bony processes listed and their positions on the skull are shown in Figure 7.3.

Although the cranium is mainly a hollowed out cavity enclosing the brain, the head itself would be too heavy to lift by the neck muscles if the bones were solid.

Consequently, several of them contain air-filled sinuses that reduce the overall weight of the head, allowing it to be held upright and looking forwards.

Table 7.1 Cranial foramina.

Bony opening	Cranial bone	Nerves and blood vessels
Carotid canal	Temporal bone	Internal carotid artery
Foramen ovale	Sphenoid bone	Mandibular division of trigeminal nerve (cranial nerve V)
Foramen rotundum	Sphenoid bone	Trigeminal nerve (cranial nerve V)
Hypoglossal canal	Occipital bone	Hypoglossal nerve (cranial nerve XII)
Internal acoustic meatus (inner ear canal)	Temporal bone	Facial nerve (cranial nerve VII) Auditory nerve (cranial nerve VIII)
Jugular foramen	Occipital and temporal bones	Internal jugular vein Glossopharyngeal nerve (cranial nerve IX) Vagus nerve (cranial nerve X) Accessory nerve (cranial nerve XI)
Stylomastoid foramen	Temporal bone	Facial nerve (cranial nerve VII)

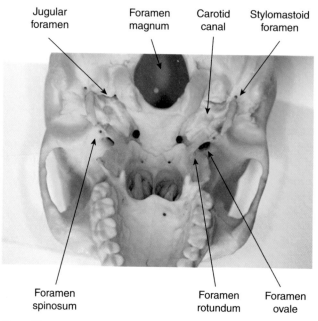

Figure 7.2 Cranial foramina.

The main cranial sinuses are as follows:

- **Frontal sinus** – in the central portion of the frontal bone, between the positions of the eyebrows
- **Mastoid process** – in the temporal bones, beneath the positions of the ears
- **Ethmoid sinus** – in the ethmoid bones, behind the nasal cavity

Table 7.2 Cranial processes.

Bony process	Cranial bone of origin	Associated structures
Mastoid process	Temporal bone	Contains air-filled spaces of the mastoid sinus and allows attachment of large neck muscle
Pterygoid process	Sphenoid bone	Extends into medial and lateral plates for attachment of muscles of mastication
Styloid process	Temporal bone	Attachment for neck muscle associated with chewing and swallowing actions
Zygomatic process	Frontal bone	Forms outer side of orbital cavities
Zygomatic process	Temporal bone	Forms portion of zygomatic arch and allows attachment of muscle of mastication

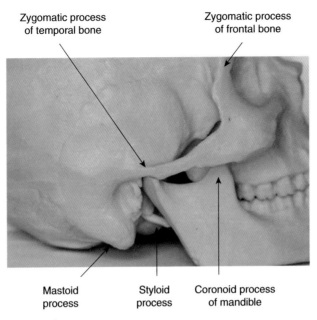

Zygomatic process
of temporal bone

Zygomatic process
of frontal bone

Mastoid
process

Styloid
process

Coronoid process
of mandible

Figure 7.3 Anatomical processes.

ANATOMY OF THE FACE

The face is composed of 14 bones that are all separated from each other by sutures, as in the cranium. The only exception is the mandible, forming the lower jaw, which articulates with the temporal bone at the hinged **temporo-mandibular joint** (TMJ).

The bones themselves are as follows:

- **Vomer** – single bone behind the nasal cavity, that articulates with cranial and other facial bones to connect the two regions of the skull together
- **Lacrimal bones** – pair of fragile bony plates forming the inner wall of the orbital cavities
- **Nasal bones** – pair of bones forming the bridge of the nose
- **Nasal turbinates** – pair of fragile curled bones projecting into the nasal cavity, which increase the contact of inspired air with the nasal mucosa – this aids debris removal before inhalation to the lungs, and warms the air
- **Palatine bones** – pair of bony plates forming the posterior section of the hard palate, and the side wall of the nasal cavity
- **Zygomatic bones** – pair of facial bones that articulate with the cranium posteriorly (frontal, temporal and sphenoid bones), and extend anteriorly into the zygomatic arch (cheek bone) to articulate with the maxilla

SKULL AND ORAL ANATOMY

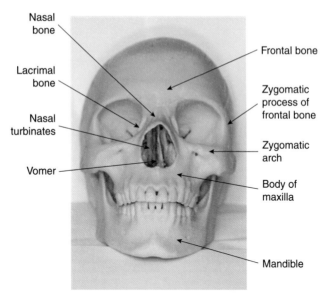

Figure 7.4 Facial bones.

- **Maxilla** – pair of bones forming the upper jaw, the lower border of the orbital cavities, the base of the nose and the anterior portion of the hard palate
- **Mandible** – single horseshoe-shaped bone forming the lower jaw, with its posterior vertical bony struts articulating with the cranium at the TMJ

The skull and facial bones are shown in Figure 7.4.

ORAL ANATOMY

The facial bones making up the oral cavity and its associated structures are of the utmost importance to all dental care professionals (DCPs). The bones will each be discussed in detail, with their associated structures covered later in this chapter.

The maxilla and palatine bones

The maxilla effectively forms the middle-third of the face, and as with various cranial bones, it has several foramina and bony projections that are dentally relevant.

The two maxilla bones join together in the centreline of the face, at the **intermaxillary suture**, and the inferior portion of these two sections form the horseshoe-shaped **alveolar process**.

It is within this process that the upper teeth form in the embryo, and later erupt as the primary then secondary dentition.

Within each half of the main body of the maxilla are the large air-filled sinuses called the **maxillary antra** (singular antrum), and the roots of the upper posterior teeth tend to be in close or intimate contact with them.

Inflammation of these air spaces (sinusitis) due to a respiratory infection often mimics dental pain in these teeth, or conversely a dental infection can be mistaken for sinusitis.

The main anatomical landmark of the maxilla from an anterior view is the **infraorbital foramen**.

This natural bony opening allows the passage of the two nerves supplying sensation to the anterior upper teeth, and their surrounding soft tissues.

Some areas and protuberances of the maxilla are also the origins of various muscles of facial expression.

The main landmarks of the maxilla from an inferior view are those of the maxillary hard palate and the alveolar process. It is here that the palatine bones are also of relevance.

The alveolar process exists purely to hold the upper teeth in situ – when the teeth are lost, the bone gradually resorbs away and the height of the process (and therefore the face) is lost permanently, unless restored by the provision of dental treatment (dentures, implants, etc.)

The palatine process of the maxilla forms the front section of the hard palate, and is fused in the midline at the **median palatine suture**. The teeth are arranged from the midline backwards on each side of the alveolar process, running from the two central incisors to the third molars.

Just palatal to the central incisors is the **incisive foramen**, where the nasopalatine nerve emerges and supplies sensation to the palatal soft tissue covering of this area.

Posterior to the third molars is a bony protuberance called the **maxillary tuberosity**, which is the very end portion of the alveolar process. It is pierced by several foramina, which allow the entry of the sensory nerve supplying the majority of the molar teeth and their buccal soft tissues.

Occasionally, a nodular enlargement of the hard palate is present, and is a benign overgrowth of bony tissue called a **palatal torus**.

The most posterior section of the hard palate is formed by the palatine bones, and with the palatine process of the maxilla they form not only the roof of the mouth, but also the floor of the nose.

The palatine bones have two foramina present, to allow entry of the sensory nerves supplying the posterior palatal soft tissues – (1) the **greater palatine foramen** and (2) the **lesser palatine foramen**.

The various anatomical landmarks of the maxilla and palatine bones are illustrated in Figures 7.5 and 7.6.

Fractures of the maxilla

From time to time, the DCP may come into contact with patients who have experienced trauma to the head and neck region. This is particularly true of

SKULL AND ORAL ANATOMY

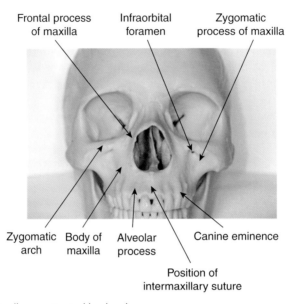

Frontal process of maxilla — Infraorbital foramen — Zygomatic process of maxilla

Zygomatic arch — Body of maxilla — Alveolar process — Canine eminence

Position of intermaxillary suture

Figure 7.5 Maxilla – anatomical landmarks.

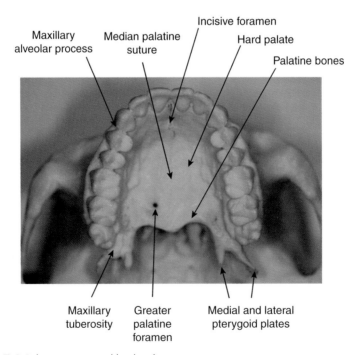

Maxillary alveolar process — Median palatine suture — Incisive foramen — Hard palate — Palatine bones

Maxillary tuberosity — Greater palatine foramen — Medial and lateral pterygoid plates

Figure 7.6 Palate – anatomical landmarks.

those working in a maxillofacial hospital department, where the management of facial trauma is one of this unit's many specialities.

Fractures of the middle-third of the face are a relatively frequent occurrence following horizontal trauma to the region, and often occur following events such as a car crash, a serious fall or a fight.

Conveniently, they have been classified into five categories ranging from the least to the most serious, as follows:

- **Alveolar fracture** – involving the anterior maxillary alveolus following a blow, or the maxillary tuberosity during tooth extraction in this region
- **Malar fracture** – involving the zygomatic arch and the surrounding bones, resulting in a fractured 'cheek bone'
- **Le Fort I fracture** – involving the separation of the palate and maxillary alveolus from the rest of the maxilla, so effectively the whole upper jaw becomes detached from the rest of the face
- **Le Fort II fracture** – involving the maxillary antrum, the nose and the base of the eye sockets, so that a pyramidal central section of the face is involved
- **Le Fort III fracture** – involving a higher fracture line through the eye sockets and the ethmoid bone behind the nose, so effectively the whole of the face becomes detached from the cranium

The Le Fort III is the most serious fracture, as the damage through the ethmoid bone effectively opens the cranium and exposes the brain to the atmosphere. The level of damage and bone displacement experienced in any maxillary fracture will depend on the force of the trauma that caused it.

The maxillary fractures are illustrated in Figure 7.7.

The mandible

The mandible is the single, horseshoe-shaped bone that forms the lower jaw, and is the only moveable bone of the skull.

Its front horizontal portion extends into the alveolar process, which holds the lower teeth in situ, while its two posterior vertical struts allow articulation with the temporal bone at the TMJ and allows the insertion at various points for the muscles of mastication.

Looking at the mandible from an anterior view, the following anatomical landmarks are visible:

- **Mental symphysis** – the fused midline point of the two halves of the mandibular processes, as they formed in the embryo
- **Mental protuberance** – the most anterior point of the bone, forming the chin
- **Mental foramen** – bony opening located between the roots of the lower premolar teeth, allowing entry of the sensory nerve supplying the

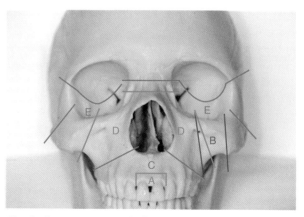

Alveolar fracture – A;   Le Fort I – C;
malar fracture of   Le Fort II – D;
cheek bone – B;   Le Fort III – E.

Figure 7.7 Maxillary fractures. A, Alveolar fracture; B, malar fracture of cheek bone; C, Le Fort I; D, Le Fort II; E, Le Fort III.

anterior teeth to the second premolar, and their buccal and labial soft tissues
- **Body of mandible** – the base of bone that supports the full length of the lower alveolar process

Figure 7.8 shows these points.

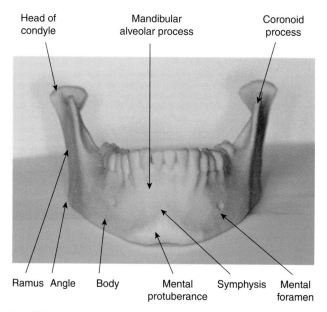

Head of condyle   Mandibular alveolar process   Coronoid process

Ramus Angle   Body   Mental protuberance   Symphysis   Mental foramen

Figure 7.8 Mandible – anterior anatomical landmarks.

Looking at the mandible from a lateral view, the following additional anatomical landmarks are visible:

- **Angle of mandible** – the corner of bone where the horizontal section turns upwards to form the vertical bony strut of the mandible
- **Ramus of mandible** – the vertical bony strut of the mandible, and the area of insertion of a muscle of mastication
- **Head of condyle** – the articulation point of the mandible with the temporal bone, at the TMJ, and the point of insertion of some muscles of mastication
- **Coronoid process** – the front bony projection of the ramus, and a point of insertion of a muscle of mastication
- **Sigmoid notch** – the dipped area between the condyle and the coronoid process, at the top of the ramus
- **Coronoid notch** – the concave anterior surface of the ramus, as it slopes to join the body of the mandible
- **External oblique line** – the crest of bone at the point where the ramus and the body join together, at the base of the coronoid notch, and the point where the **long buccal nerve** crosses from the lateral surface of the body to the medial surface, carrying sensory nerves from the buccal soft tissues of the lower molar teeth

Figure 7.9 shows these points.

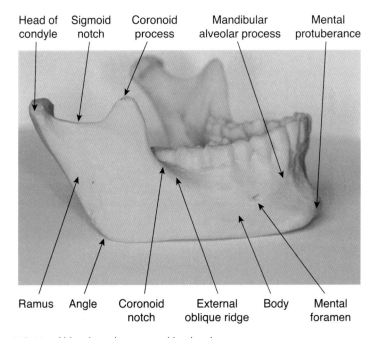

Figure 7.9 Mandible – lateral anatomical landmarks.

SKULL AND ORAL ANATOMY

Looking at the mandible from a medial view, the following anatomical landmarks are visible:

- **Genial tubercles** – bony projections around the midline point of the medial surface of the body, and the point of insertion of various of the suprahyoid muscles
- **Mylohyoid ridge** – bony line running horizontally along the medial surface of the body, and the point of attachment of the mylohyoid muscle that forms the floor of the mouth
- **Sublingual fossa** – shallow depression above the mylohyoid ridge anteriorly, where the sublingual salivary gland sits
- **Submandibular fossa** – shallow depression below the mylohyoid ridge posteriorly, where the submandibular salivary gland sits
- **Retromolar triangle** – roughened posterior end of the alveolar process, posterior to the third molar, where a thickened soft tissue covering forms the retromolar pad
- **Mandibular foramen** – bony opening on the medial surface of the ramus, where the sensory inferior dental (ID) nerve exits the mandible and travels to the central nervous system
- **Lingula** – protective bony projection that lies across the front edge of the mandibular foramen

Figure 7.10 shows these points.

SKULL AND ORAL ANATOMY

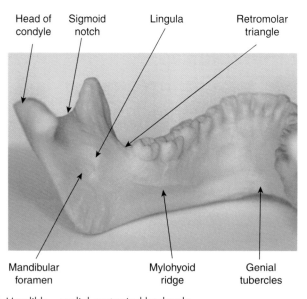

Head of condyle   Sigmoid notch   Lingula   Retromolar triangle

Mandibular foramen   Mylohyoid ridge   Genial tubercles

Figure 7.10 Mandible – medial anatomical landmarks.

Occasionally, bilateral nodular enlargements of the anterior area of the medial surface of the body of the mandible are present, and are benign overgrowths of bony tissue called **mandibular tori**.

Fractures of the mandible

As with the maxilla, the mandible can also be fractured following trauma to the lower face, including that experienced during a difficult tooth extraction.

Although not classified, there are five common areas of mandibular fracture that may occur, as follows:

- **Alveolar fracture** – involving the anterior mandibular alveolus when due to trauma, although it can occur anywhere along the alveolar process during tooth extraction
- **Canine region fracture** – involving the body of the mandible in this region following one-sided trauma, and occurring here due to the relative bony weakness produced by the large canine tooth socket
- **Midline fracture** – involving the mental symphysis and often following a blow to the chin, effectively splitting the mandible into its two halves
- **Angle fracture** – involving the separation of the ramus of the mandible from the body on the side of the trauma, and occurring here due to the relative bony weakness produced by the third molar socket
- **Condylar fracture** – involving one or both of the condyles, following a blow to the opposite side of the jaw or to the chin with the mouth open, respectively

Unlike the maxilla, the level of bony displacement following mandibular fracture depends on the pull of both the muscles of mastication and the suprahyoids.

Displacement is often extensive and requires surgery to pin, wire and plate the bone ends together again. In some circumstances, the bony displacement may enable the tongue to fall back and compromise the airway.

Mandibular fractures often result in derangement of the occlusion, as the bone ends and their teeth are pulled out of line with each other.

The mandibular fractures are illustrated in Figure 7.11.

The temporomandibular joint

The TMJs are the bilateral joints between the mandible and the cranium that allow mouth closure, and jaw movements during speech and mastication.

Mouth opening occurs due to the action of some of the suprahyoid muscles.

The joint is formed where the head of condyle of the mandible sits in a depression in the under surface of the temporal bone, called the **glenoid fossa,** to form a hinged arrangement.

The two bones are separated by a cartilage disc called the **meniscus,** which prevents the bones from grating together during joint movement.

SKULL AND ORAL ANATOMY

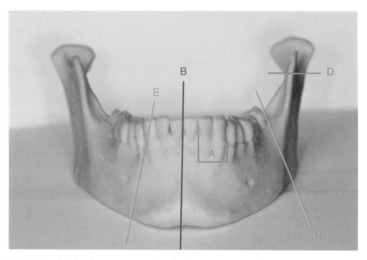

Figure 7.11 Mandibular fractures. A, Alveolar fracture; B, midline fracture; C, angle fracture; D, condyle fracture; E, canine region fracture.

The disc and both bony areas of the joint are intricately held together by the **muscles of mastication,** and their associated tendons and ligaments.

The anterior surface of the glenoid fossa extends into a prominent, rounded bony ridge called the **articular eminence**. This structure helps to prevent jaw dislocation during normal joint movements, as the condyle head does not normally move anterior to this landmark.

Figure 7.12 illustrates the arrangement of the TMJ.

During normal jaw movements, the joint allows three basic types of mandibular movement to occur:

- **Gliding movement** – mainly occurs when the disc and the condyle together slide up and down the articular eminence, allowing the mandible to move forwards and backwards (protrusion and retraction, respectively)
- **Rotational movement** – occurs when the condyle rotates anteriorly and posteriorly over the surface of the disc itself, which remains static, allowing the mandible to move down and up (depression and elevation, respectively)
- **Lateral movement** – this occurs when one joint glides alone, so that the other condyle rotates sideways over its disc

The actions of the muscles of mastication during these movements are explained later in this chapter.

The resting position of the TMJ is such that the teeth are slightly out of contact between the jaws, so that a natural space is present between the occlusal surfaces. This natural space is normally around 2 mm, and is called the **freeway space.**

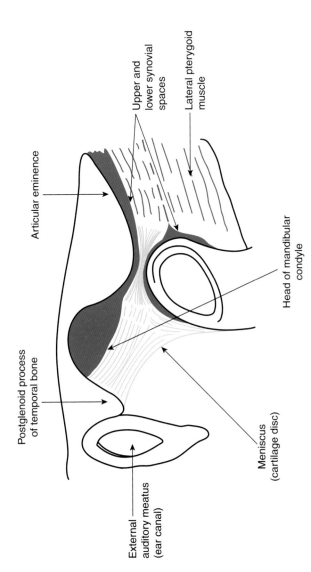

Figure 7.12 Temporomandibular joint arrangement.

Articular eminence

Upper and lower synovial spaces

Lateral pterygoid muscle

Postglenoid process of temporal bone

Head of mandibular condyle

External auditory meatus (ear canal)

Meniscus (cartilage disc)

SKULL AND ORAL ANATOMY

During the placement of dental restorations and prostheses, it is imperative that the freeway space is maintained, otherwise the joint will be forced to do one of the following actions:

- Open further than it should to clear a premature contact, causing muscle strain around the joint
- Over close to achieve occlusion, causing muscle strain and facial discomfort

Both situations will be extremely uncomfortable for the patient.

Disorders of the TMJ

As with any joint, the TMJs can be affected by **osteoarthritis** and require the use of anti-inflammatories or steroids to relieve the painful symptoms.

In extreme cases involving younger patients, the joints can even be replaced by artificial prostheses, as with hips and knees.

Parafunctional habits of the patient, especially habitual clenching and grinding of the teeth over long periods, tends to exhaust the joint musculature and cause pain and discomfort.

This action is called **bruxism**, and most patients are unaware that they perform these habitual movements, often doing so in their sleep.

Sufferers will experience any or all of the following symptoms:

- **Trismus** – involuntary painful contracture of the joint musculature, resulting in the inability to open the mouth fully
- **Face and/or neck pain** – often worse in the morning following a night of bruxing, and eased by relaxation and the use of anti-inflammatories
- **Attrition** – wear facets on the teeth, due to the constant wearing of the occlusal and incisal surfaces of each arch against the other
- **Restorative failure** – repetitive fracture and loss of dental restorations, with or without tooth fracture, due to the excessive and prolonged occlusal forces produced
- **Sore mouth** – especially the tongue and cheeks, where cheek ridges and tongue scalloping develop as the tongue is thrust against the teeth, and the cheeks are bitten

Similar symptoms are often seen in patients who use chewing gum excessively.

Following diagnosis and advice on the particular cause of the bruxism, which can often be in relation to stress, treatment involves counselling, use of anti-inflammatories and muscle relaxants and sometimes the provision of night guards or splints to wear as necessary.

While not preventing the bruxing action, these devices will hold the jaws open slightly and relieve the tension put on the joint musculature.

In some cases, life changes may be necessary.

Temporomandibular dysfunction occurs when there is a derangement of the disc within the joint capsule.

In its mildest forms, it can exhibit as occasional joint popping and clicking on opening and closing the mouth. In more severe cases, one of the following may occur:

- **Subluxation** – the disc becomes displaced so that the joint surfaces are not fully in correct contact with each other
- **Dislocation** – the joint is badly disrupted, and the joint surfaces are fully out of correct contact with each other

Subluxation usually occurs on excessive mouth opening (especially when yawning or opening too wide when biting), and the mandible needs manipulating down and backwards to align the joint again. This may require the use of muscle relaxants such as low doses of benzodiazepines first.

Dislocation is usually associated with trauma, including the use of prolonged and excessive force during a lower tooth extraction, by the dentist. These cases require referral to the oral and maxillofacial department for treatment.

Temporomandibular disorder

This is a more difficult condition to diagnose, as the sufferer can experience a wide range of non-specific symptoms, including:

- Swelling over the TMJ region
- Chronic tenderness of the TMJ
- Difficulty in performing normal TMJ movements
- Spasms of the joint musculature
- Joint derangement with joint sounds
- Facial pain
- Head, neck and back pain
- Other chronic body pain

The diagnosis and management of these patients is complicated, and beyond the remit of this text.

MUSCLES

The musculature of the skull is of importance to the DCP, to enable understanding of the complicated activities involved in mastication, speech and swallowing.

The groups of muscles to be discussed are as follows:

- Muscles of mastication
- Suprahyoid muscles
- Muscles of facial expression
- Tongue

SKULL AND ORAL ANATOMY

Muscles of mastication

These muscles are of the skeletal type, so by definition they are responsible for the movement of bones.

They are arranged as a group of four paired muscles, attached between the cranium and the mandible, and are responsible for mouth closing and chewing movements of the mandible.

The four pairs are:

- Temporalis muscles
- Masseter muscles
- Medial pterygoid muscles
- Lateral pterygoid muscles

All of the muscles of mastication are innervated by the motor branch of the mandibular division of the trigeminal nerve (cranial nerve V).

As discussed in Chapter 1, skeletal muscles carry out their actions by being attached at either end to different bones and contracting, so that the length of muscle is shortened.

This muscle shortening will then move one bone towards the other, the insertion to the origin, to produce the action of the muscle.

Temporalis muscles

- Point of origin – in a fan shape over the surface of the temporal bone of the cranium
- Point of insertion – coronoid process of the mandible
- Action – full muscle contraction lifts the mandible and closes the jaw in a **rotational** movement, posterior contraction only pulls the jaw backwards in a **gliding** movement

Masseter muscles

- Point of origin – superficial (outer) fibres from the front section of the zygomatic arch, deep (inner) fibres from the back section and inner surface of the zygomatic arch
- Point of insertion – superficial fibres to the outer surface of the angle of the mandible, deep fibres to the outer surface of the ramus of the mandible
- Action – lifts the mandible and closes the jaw in a **rotational** movement

Medial pterygoid muscles

- Point of origin – medial pterygoid plate of the sphenoid bone of the cranium
- Point of insertion – inner surface of the ramus of the mandible
- Action – lifts the mandible and closes the jaw in a **rotational** movement

Temporal muscle

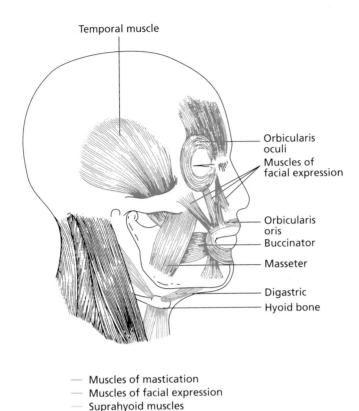

Orbicularis
oculi

Muscles of
facial expression

Orbicularis
oris

Buccinator

Masseter

Digastric

Hyoid bone

— Muscles of mastication
— Muscles of facial expression
— Suprahyoid muscles

Figure 7.13 Oral musculature. (From Hollins, C. (2008). *Levison's Textbook for Dental Nurses*, 10th edn. Blackwell Publishing, Oxford. Reproduced with permission from John Wiley & Sons, Ltd.)

Lateral pterygoid muscles

- Point of origin – superior (upper) fibres from the sphenoid bone of the cranium, inferior (lower) fibres from the lateral pterygoid plate of the sphenoid bone
- Point of insertion – most superior fibres run into the TMJ capsule, all other fibres to the anterior (front) surface of the condyle of the mandible
- Action – both sides contracting moves the jaw forwards so the incisor teeth are tip to tip in a **gliding** movement, if one side contracts the jaw swings sideways to the opposite side in a **lateral** movement

The locations of the muscles of mastication are shown in Figure 7.13.

Suprahyoid muscles

Again, these muscles are of the skeletal type and are connected to bone and other structures in the neck.

As their name suggests, one end of all these muscles is attached to the horseshoe-shaped **hyoid bone** that lies suspended in soft tissue beneath the mandible, in the throat. They then all lie above the bone, as opposed to a separate group of muscles lying beneath the bone called the **infrahyoid muscles**.

The suprahyoid muscles are responsible for mouth opening and swallowing actions.

One group of muscles lie in front of the hyoid bone, and the others behind, producing anterior and posterior groups, respectively.

They are:

- Anterior group – anterior digastric, mylohyoid and geniohyoid muscles
- Posterior group – posterior digastric and stylohyoid muscles

The anterior digastric and mylohyoid muscles are innervated by the motor branch of the trigeminal nerve (cranial nerve V).

The geniohyoid muscle is partly innervated by the hypoglossal nerve (cranial nerve XII).

The posterior digastric and stylohyoid muscles are innervated by the facial nerve (cranial nerve VII).

Digastric muscles

- Point of origin – anterior, hyoid bone; posterior, mastoid region of the temporal bone
- Point of insertion – anterior, inner surface of mental symphysis of the mandible; posterior, hyoid bone
- Action – anterior and posterior lift the hyoid bone and larynx during swallowing, anterior only pulls the jaw down to open the mouth

Mylohyoid muscles

- Point of origin – mylohyoid line of the inner surface of the mandible, fusing in the midline to form the floor of the mouth
- Point of insertion – hyoid bone
- Action – lift hyoid bone and larynx during swallowing, and open the mouth

Geniohyoid muscles

- Point of origin – genial tubercles on inner surface of the mandible
- Point of insertion – hyoid bone
- Action – lift hyoid bone and larynx during swallowing, and open the mouth

Stylohyoid muscles

- Point of origin – styloid process of the temporal bone
- Point of insertion – hyoid bone
- Action – lift the hyoid bone and larynx during swallowing

The locations of the suprahyoid muscles are shown in Figure 7.13.

SKULL AND ORAL ANATOMY

Muscles of facial expression

These are the muscles concerned with actioning the numerous facial expressions that humans are capable of exhibiting.

In contrast to the muscles of mastication, those of facial expression are not involved in producing skeletal movement and most are only attached at one end to the skull. Their other ends are inserted into the deep layer of the facial skin only, so that their contraction causes skin movement only.

All of the muscles of facial expression are innervated by the motor branch of the facial nerve (cranial nerve VII).

They can be grouped according to the facial region that their actions involve:

- The scalp
- The eyes and surrounding area
- The mouth and surrounding area

The last group only are of interest to the DCP.

The group consists of 12 pairs of muscles around the mouth region, and it is beyond the requirement of DCPs to name and describe them all.

For the sake of completeness, the 12 pairs are listed in Table 7.3, but only those in bold are of concern in this text.

The locations of some of the muscles of facial expression are shown in Figure 7.13.

The tongue

The tongue is a muscular organ situated in the oral cavity and the throat.

The posterior section, the **base of the tongue**, lies in the throat and attaches to the floor of the mouth.

It is relatively firmly attached and is mainly concerned with swallowing movements.

The correct term for swallowing is **deglutition**.

The remaining anterior two-thirds of the tongue, the **body**, lie within the oral cavity and this section is relatively moveable, being able to perform numerous convoluted movements.

It is concerned with taste, chewing activities and speech.

The role of the tongue in determining taste sensation is described in Chapter 6.

The organ is composed of symmetrical muscular halves joined at the fibrous midpoint along its length.

The midpoint corresponds visibly to the central groove of the dorsal surface of the body, called the **median lingual sulcus**.

The gross anatomy of the tongue is shown in Figure 7.14.

The muscles of the tongue are divided into two basic groups – the **intrinsic muscles** and the **extrinsic muscles**.

SKULL AND ORAL ANATOMY

Table 7.3 Muscles of facial expression.

Name	Origin	Insertion	Action
Orbicularis oris	**Soft tissues surrounding the oral cavity**	**Skin tissue at the angle of the mouth**	**Shapes and controls the size of the opening to the oral cavity**
Buccinator	**Alveolar processes (vertical fibres) and regional soft tissues (horizontal fibres)**	**Skin tissue at the angle of the mouth**	**Forms the cheek Assists with chewing actions**
Mentalis	**Midline of mandible**	**Skin tissue of the chin**	**Narrows the oral opening by raising the chin tissue**
Depressor anguli oris	Lower border of mandible	Skin tissue at the angle of the mouth	Pulls mouth corners down – frowning
Depressor labii inferioris	Lower border of mandible	Skin tissue of lower lip	Pulls lower lip down
Levator anguli oris	Canine region of maxilla	Skin tissue at the angle of the mouth	Raises corners of mouth – smiling
Risorius	Soft tissues over masseter muscle	Skin tissue at the angle of the mouth	Widens the oral opening
Levator labii superioris (LLS)	Infraorbital rim of maxilla	Skin tissue of upper lip	Raises upper lip
LLS alaeque nasi	Front of maxilla	Skin tissues of nostrils and upper lip	Raises upper lip and flares nostrils
Zygomaticus major	Zygomatic bone	Skin tissue at the angle of the mouth	Smiling
Zygomaticus minor	Zygomatic bone	Skin tissue of upper lip	Smiling
Platysma	Skin tissue over shoulder and collar bone	Lower border of mandible	Pulls corner of mouth down Raises skin of the neck

All are innervated by the hypoglossal nerve (cranial nerve XII).

The intrinsic muscles lie within the body of the tongue entirely, and are responsible for the following movements:

- Shortening and thickening the organ
- Curling the edges
- Curling the tip
- Lengthening and narrowing it

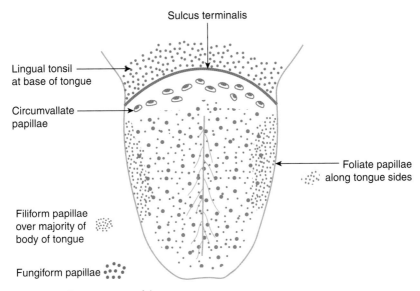

Figure 7.14 Gross anatomy of the tongue.

Besides speech, these movements are required to assist the buccinator muscles to shape and roll ingested food particles into a small sausage-like shape called a food bolus.

The extrinsic muscles all have origins outside the tongue, and insertions within it, as shown in Table 7.4.

Once the food bolus is formed, the body and base of the tongue act together with the muscles of the soft palate, the pharynx and the suprahyoids to guide the bolus backwards and perform the swallowing action.

The swallowing action occurs as follows:

- Body of the tongue moves the bolus to the back of the oral cavity – the oropharynx
- Soft palate muscles raise the soft palate posteriorly to seal the nasal cavity from the oral cavity

Table 7.4 Extrinsic muscles of the tongue.

Name	Origin	Insertion	Action
Genioglossus	Genial tubercles of the mandible	Ventral surface of the full tongue	Tongue protrusion Tongue depression
Hyoglossus	Hyoid bone	Lateral surface of the body	Tongue depression
Styloglossus	Styloid process of temporal bone	Tongue apex Junction of body and base	Tongue retraction

SKULL AND ORAL ANATOMY

- Pharyngeal muscles assist in sealing off the nasal cavity
- Base of tongue guides the bolus into the pharynx
- Suprahyoid muscles raise the larynx and hyoid bone, allowing the epiglottis to drop down and seal off the trachea, preventing food inhalation
- Pharyngeal muscles constrict to push the bolus past the epiglottis and into the opening of the oesophagus
- Peristaltic action of the oesophagus moves the bolus down towards the stomach

The event is illustrated in Figure 7.15.

This complicated swallowing action is voluntarily controllable up to the point where the bolus passes backwards from the oral cavity; from this point onwards the bolus is either involuntarily swallowed or expelled forcefully from the pharynx by the act of coughing.

The four sets of muscles involved in swallowing are in total innervated by cranial nerves V, IX, X, XI and XII, an indication of the complexity of the actions involved in what may be considered as a straightforward bodily function.

The condition of **dysphagia**, or difficulty in swallowing, occurs relatively frequently and has several causes:

- Psychological – an inability to swallow (invariably) medication in tablet form, although food and drink can be swallowed normally
- Xerostomia – dry mouth syndrome, where reduced salivary flow prevents adequate bolus lubrication
- Oesophagitis – often due to acid reflux
- Other conditions affecting pharyngeal or oesophageal function, including cancers
- CNS disorders preventing correct muscle innervation, such as stroke and multiple sclerosis

NERVE SUPPLY TO THE ORAL CAVITY

The numerous cranial nerves innervating the head and neck region have been mentioned in various areas of the text, and this section will concentrate on the detail of the nerve supply to the oral cavity itself.

The two cranial nerves of key importance to the DCP are:

- **Trigeminal nerve** – cranial nerve V
- **Facial nerve** – cranial nerve VII

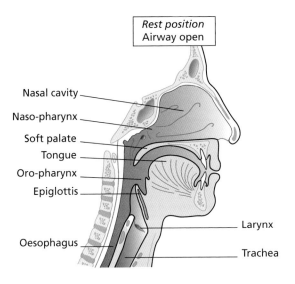

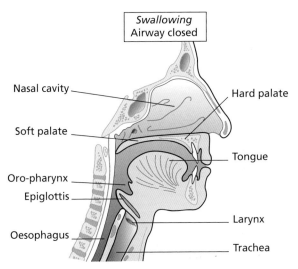

Figure 7.15 Swallowing action. (From Hollins, C. (2008). *Levison's Textbook for Dental Nurses*, 10th edn. Blackwell Publishing, Oxford. Reproduced with permission from John Wiley & Sons, Ltd.)

Trigeminal nerve

This cranial nerve is so called because its main trunk within the cranium is composed of three separate divisions:

- Ophthalmic division
- Maxillary division
- Mandibular division

SKULL AND ORAL ANATOMY

All three divisions are composed of sensory nerves that carry sensation from their respective areas of innervation, and the mandibular division also carries motor nerves from the brain to the muscles of mastication.

The maxillary and mandibular divisions are of the greatest importance to the DCP, as they directly supply the structures of the oral cavity.

As with all nerves throughout the body, these divisions can each be imagined as the main trunk of a tree, which then sub-divides to form various branches, which are then each named as separate nerves. These often go on to sub-divide further into smaller and smaller nerves themselves.

To understand the complexity of the nerve supply to the oral cavity, the DCP not only needs to know the names of the relevant branches and their area of innervation, but also the path that they take through the oral tissues on their journey to and/or from the brain.

In accordance with usual anatomical terminology, nerves tend to be named after the area they supply and, with the addition of positional terms to describe where they originate, the final title of each nerve will state exactly their relationship to the surrounding structures.

So, for example the anterior superior dental nerve originates at the front portion of the upper alveolar region (the maxilla), from the teeth and their surrounding tissues.

Maxillary division

The division originates from five branches, one of which has two further sub-branches (Figure 7.16).

The maxillary nerve enters the cranium through the **foramen rotundum**.

The **zygomatic nerve** carries sensory nerve impulses from the skin in this region, and is of no dental relevance.

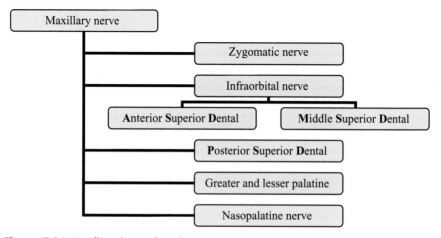

Figure 7.16 Maxillary division branches.

The **infraorbital nerve (IO nerve)** is made up of the sensory sub-branches from the anterior and middle sections of the upper alveolar process, which run from the pulp tissue of the relevant teeth, and their associated periodontal tissues and labial/buccal gingivae.

The anterior superior dental (ASD) nerve details are:

- Sensation from upper incisors and canine teeth, their periodontium and labial gingivae
- Pathway up through the maxillary antrum to join the IO nerve

The middle superior dental (MSD) nerve details are:

- Sensation from upper premolar teeth and the mesiobuccal root of the first molar, their periodontium and buccal gingivae
- Pathway along the side wall of the maxillary antrum to join the IO nerve

The IO nerve details are:

- Sensation from the infraorbital skin region and upper lip
- Pathway through the infraorbital foramen into the IO canal, where it is joined by ASD and MSD nerves

The posterior superior dental (PSD) nerve details are:

- Sensation from the upper molar teeth (except the mesiobuccal (MB) root of 6s), their periodontium and buccal gingivae and the membranes of the maxillary sinus
- Pathway out of the antrum in the region of the maxillary tuberosity, and travels up to join the IO nerve as it leaves the IO canal, behind the maxilla

The **greater palatine nerve** details are:

- Sensation from the palatal gingivae of the upper premolar and molar teeth, and the soft tissues over the adjacent hard palate
- Pathway off the hard palate through the greater palatine foramen, and up between the pterygoid plates to join the maxillary nerve

The **lesser palatine nerve** details are:

- Sensation from the soft palate and tonsils
- Pathway out of the oral cavity through the lesser palatine foramen and joins the greater palatine nerve route

The **nasopalatine nerve** details are:

- Sensation from the palatal gingivae of the upper incisors and canine teeth, and the soft tissues over the adjacent hard palate
- Pathway out of the oral cavity through the incisive foramen, then along the nasal septum to join the maxillary nerve

The nasopalatine nerve is sometimes referred to as the long sphenopalatine nerve.

The maxillary division branches are illustrated in Figure 7.17.

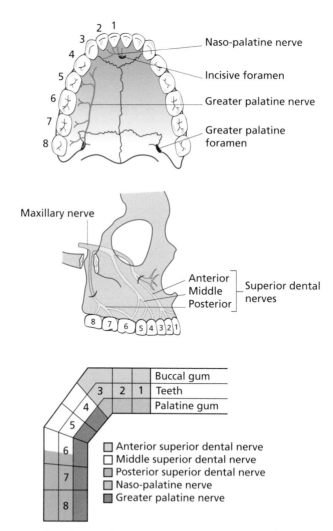

Figure 7.17 Maxillary division of trigeminal nerve. (From Hollins, C. (2008). *Levison's Textbook for Dental Nurses*, 10th edn. Blackwell Publishing, Oxford. Reproduced with permission from John Wiley & Sons, Ltd.)

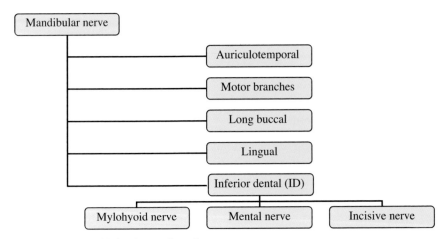

Figure 7.18 Mandibular division branches.

Mandibular division

The division originates from five branches, one of which has three further sub-branches (Figure 7.18).

The **auriculotemporal nerve** carries sensory nerve impulses from the skin around the ear and the scalp in this region.

It also carries parasympathetic fibres to the parotid salivary gland, acting to reduce salivary flow to a normal 'post-food' level.

The **motor branches** travel from the brain and out of the cranium through the **foramen ovale,** carrying motor impulses to the muscles of mastication.

The **long buccal nerve** details are:

- Sensation from the buccal gingivae of the lower molar teeth, the adjacent buccal mucosa and the skin of the cheek
- Pathway from the adjacent buccal sulcus region and across the retromolar region to join the mandibular nerve deep to the pterygoid muscles

The **lingual nerve** details are:

- Sensation from the lingual gingivae of all the lower teeth, the floor of the mouth and the body of the tongue (**not taste**)
- Pathway from these regions posteriorly and then ascends the inner surface of the ramus of the mandible to join the mandibular nerve

The **inferior dental nerve** is made up of the sensory sub-branches of the mental and incisive nerves, which receive sensation from all of the lower teeth.

It also has a motor sub-branch (the mylohyoid nerve) that innervates the mylohyoid and anterior digastric muscles of the suprahyoids. This splits from the ID nerve just as it exits the mandible through the mandibular foramen.

The incisive nerve details are:

- Sensation from the lower anterior and premolar teeth, and their associated periodontal tissues
- Pathway from the anterior region of the outer surface of the mandible, posteriorly to join the mental nerve at the mental foramen

The mental nerve details are:

- Sensation from the skin of the chin and lower lip, and the labial and buccal mucosa of the lower anterior teeth to the second premolar
- Pathway from these regions posteriorly to enter the mandible at the mental foramen, with the incisive nerve

The ID nerve details are:

- Sensation from all regions supplied by the incisive and mental sub-branches
- Pathway posteriorly through the mandibular canal from the mental foramen, to exit the mandible through the mandibular foramen on the inner surface of the ramus, then to join the mandibular nerve

The mandibular division branches are illustrated in Figure 7.19.

Trigeminal neuralgia

This is a condition affecting the sensory nerves of either the maxillary or mandibular divisions only of the trigeminal nerve, with no known cause.

The sufferer experiences sudden onset, severe pain in various facial trigger zones, accompanied by muscle spasms in the area.

The neuralgia can be initiated by touch, chewing movements or even speaking, and are usually of short duration. Treatment is difficult without a known cause, and often drastic measures such as the surgical or chemical destruction of the sensory section of the nerve is undertaken, to relieve the debilitating symptoms.

Facial nerve

As the name suggests, this cranial nerve is so named because it supplies various structures in the facial region of the skull.

It contains both sensory and motor divisions, but the names of all of the various branches are of little relevance to the DCP. Only the most important ones will be discussed here.

The nerve divides into two main divisions within the cranium, and then proceeds as follows:

- **Motor** and **parasympathetic division**, which leaves through the internal acoustic meatus
- **Motor division**, which leaves through the stylomastoid foramen

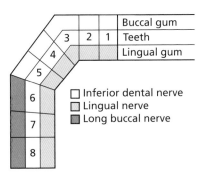

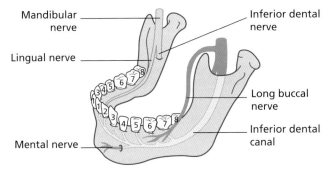

Figure 7.19 Mandibular division of trigeminal nerve. (From Hollins, C. (2008). *Levison's Textbook for Dental Nurses*, 10th edn. Blackwell Publishing, Oxford. Reproduced with permission from John Wiley & Sons, Ltd.)

Internal acoustic meatus branches

Motor branch travels to the tiny bones within the middle ear (the ear ossicles), which are involved in the sensation of hearing.

Parasympathetic branches run as two nerves:

- **Chorda tympani nerve**
  - To the submandibular and sublingual salivary glands, to increase salivary flow
  - Taste sensation from the anterior two-third of the tongue
- **Greater petrosal nerve**
  - To the minor salivary glands of the palate
  - Taste sensation from the palate

Stylomastoid foramen branches

These are all motor branches and supply the following:

- **Posterior auricular nerve** – facial expression muscles of the scalp
- **Posterior suprahyoid branches** – stylohyoid muscle and posterior digastric muscle

- **Terminal branches within the parotid gland** – all other muscles of facial expression

Bell's palsy

This is a condition of uncertain origin that affects the facial nerve on one side. The sufferer experiences sudden onset one-sided facial paralysis, affecting some or all of the muscles of facial expression. The 'sagging face' appearance may mimic the after-effects of a stroke in severe cases.

The condition usually clears itself, or can become chronic if the nerve transmission of the facial nerve is badly compromised.

Facial paralysis, due to traumatic injury or disease and surgery in the region of the parotid gland, will often produce a similar facial appearance, as the facial nerve travels intimately through this structure.

BLOOD SUPPLY TO THE HEAD AND NECK REGION

The circulatory system of the body was discussed in detail in Chapter 2, and the supply of the oral cavity follows the general format described:

- Oxygenated blood supplies the area via arteries and their smaller branches, from the left side of the heart
- Deoxygenated blood is removed from the area by veins and their smaller branches, to the right side of the heart
- Lymph vessels collect additional tissue fluid present, and return it to the circulatory system

The blood vessels involved tend to run alongside the nerves of the area, as **neurovascular bundles**. This arrangement tends to occur throughout the body, and ensures that the vessels can be more easily located than if they all ran along their own courses. Similarly, they may also enter and leave the bony cavities of the skull through the same foramina and fissures.

The names of the various blood vessels of the oral cavity are not required knowledge for DCPs, but they tend to follow the nerve nomenclature covered previously by being named after their area of supply, as a general rule.

So the artery supplying the maxillary portion of the face is, unsurprisingly, the **maxillary artery**, while the vein associated with the same area is the **maxillary vein**, and so on.

Arterial blood supply

The major arteries carrying oxygenated blood to the head and neck region are the **common carotid arteries**, which are direct branches from the arch of the aorta as it leaves the left ventricle.

These travel up the left and right sides of the neck, and are palpable against either side of the larynx as the **carotid pulse**, often taken during medical emergencies and CPR.

Around this position, the common carotids divide into the following major arteries:

- **External carotid artery** – supplying all of the head outside of the cranium, including the face and the oral cavity
- **Internal carotid artery** – supplying all of the inner cranial structures including the brain, and the eyes

Further detail of the inner carotid artery is outside the remit of this text.

The four main branches of the external carotid artery sub-divide further still, and their end branches are numerous. The sub-branches of particular interest to the DCP are highlighted in Table 7.5.

Table 7.5 Carotid artery sub-branches.

Main branch	Sub-branches	Areas of supply
Anterior	Superior thyroid	Neck muscles
	Lingual	**Floor of mouth** **Tongue** **Sublingual salivary gland**
	Facial	**Soft tissues of facial region** **Submandibular salivary gland** **Some muscles of facial expression** **Some suprahyoid muscles**
Medial	Ascending pharyngeal	Soft palate Pharyngeal walls Brain meninges
Posterior	Occipital	Neck muscles Scalp Brain meninges
	Posterior auricular	Internal ear Mastoid process
Terminal	**Superficial temporal**	**Parotid salivary gland** Portions of scalp
	Maxillary	**Maxillary teeth** **Mandibular teeth** **Soft tissues of oral cavity** **Muscles of mastication** **Buccinator muscle** **Hard and soft palates** **Nasal cavity** Brain meninges

SKULL AND ORAL ANATOMY

Diagrammatically, the blood supply to the head and neck region follows the pathways of the nerve supply to the region, within the neurovascular bundles referred to previously.

Venous drainage

Once the usual gaseous exchange has occurred in the capillary beds of the head and neck region, deoxygenated blood tends to flow from small venules into gradually widening veins, until they reach the main venous vessels of the area:

- **External jugular vein** – draining a small area of extracranial tissues only
- **Internal jugular vein** – draining the brain and the majority of the head and neck tissues

The names of the various smaller drainage vessels are of little importance to the DCP, and tend to mirror those of the arterial supply anyway. So, the area supplied by the facial artery is drained by the facial vein, and so on.

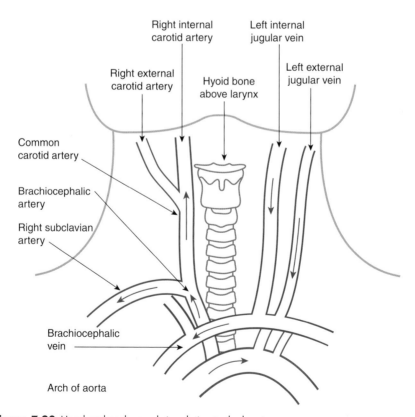

Figure 7.20 Head and neck vessels in relation to the heart.

The small external jugular vein and the larger internal jugular vein, join the major vessels draining the arms and the surrounding areas – the **subclavian veins**.

These then run into the **brachiocephalic veins**, which join together to become the **superior vena cava**, which returns all blood from the upper body to the right atrium of the heart.

The major blood vessels of the head and neck are shown in diagrammatic relationship to the heart in Figure 7.20.

The flow of deoxygenated blood from the head and neck region is not always in one direction, as occurs in other areas of the body. This is because the veins of this area usually do not contain the one-way valve system present in the majority of these vessels, so blood can flow forwards and backwards depending on changes affecting the local pressure.

Generally then, it is easier for localised infections to spread in the head and neck regions than elsewhere in the body. The seriousness of this statement is compounded further by the fact that the blood travels through the most important organ of the body, the brain, and that pathogens may enter the area in a variety of ways:

- Inhaled through the nose or mouth
- Ingested through the oral cavity
- Carried by the circulatory or lymph systems
- Traumatically deposited through the soft tissues; during dental treatment, local anaesthetic (LA) injection or head and neck injury

The need for the maintenance of high standards of infection control in the field of dentistry is therefore of paramount importance, and of great concern to the whole oral health care team.

SKULL AND ORAL ANATOMY

Chapter 8

Tooth anatomy

Tooth embryology and eruption are discussed in Chapter 7.

THE TOOTH – GROSS ANATOMY

Although the permanent dentition is made up of four morphologically different types of teeth, the gross anatomy of each is the same. Their shape, or morphology, differs depending on their function and this will be discussed later.

The four types, from the midline to posterior, are:

- Central and lateral incisors
- Canine
- First and second premolars
- First, second and third molars

The primary dentition (also referred to as the deciduous dentition) is made up of just three different types of teeth – there are no premolars present. The differences between the two dentitions is summarised later.

Each tooth has three sections, (1) the **crown**, (2) the **neck** and (3) the **root**.

The crown is the section of the tooth visible in the oral cavity, following its eruption from the underlying alveolar bone. The neck is the section where the tooth and the gingival tissues are in contact with each other, and the root is the (usually) non-visible section that holds the tooth in its bony socket.

All teeth are composed of the same four tissues:

- **Enamel** – covering the whole crown of the tooth
- **Dentine** – forming the inner bulk of the crown and root
- **Cementum** – a thin covering of the root dentine only
- **Pulp** – the inner neurovascular tissue of the tooth, within the central pulp chamber

The gross anatomy of the tooth is shown in Figure 8.1.

Basic Guide to Anatomy and Physiology for Dental Care Professionals, First Edition. Carole Hollins.
© 2012 John Wiley & Sons, Ltd. Published 2012 by John Wiley & Sons, Ltd.

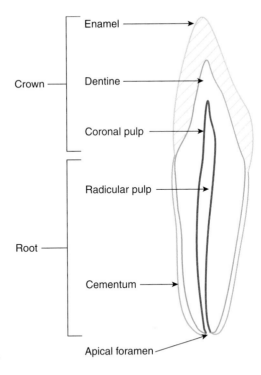

Enamel

Dentine

Crown

Coronal pulp

Radicular pulp

Root

Cementum

Apical foramen

Figure 8.1 Gross anatomy of a tooth.

THE TOOTH – MICROSCOPIC ANATOMY AND HISTOLOGY

Early enamel and dentine

The outer surface of the crown of the tooth, enamel, is derived embryologically from the ectoderm layer of the early foetus, as the enamel organ.

The inner bulk of the tooth, dentine, is derived embryologically from the specialised neuroectoderm layer, and these two layers are separated by the basement membrane.

Differentiation of the embryological tissues of the tooth begins at around 6 weeks after conception.

Full details of the embryological development of the teeth are given in Chapter 7.

Once the developing tooth has reached the bell stage, the final two stages that occur result in the formation of the tooth as it appears on eruption into the oral cavity. These two stages are:

- **Apposition** – the enamel, dentine and cementum are laid down layer upon layer, initially as a partially calcified matrix
- **Maturation** – the enamel, dentine and cementum become fully mineralised

TOOTH ANATOMY

The matrix formed during apposition is secreted out of the cells into the surrounding area, and is partly calcified so that it can act as the crystalline frame on which future mineralisation can occur, during maturation.

At the bell stage, the innermost layer of epithelial cells of the enamel organ line up along the basement membrane, at the same time as the outermost layer of the underlying dental papilla lines up on the inner side of the basement membrane.

The enamel organ cells then differentiate into **ameloblasts**, while the dental papilla cells differentiate into **odontoblasts**.

The process of **dentinogenesis** now begins, where the odontoblasts lay down layers of dentine matrix between themselves and the basement membrane, so that the cells gradually move away from the basement membrane.

This cell activity causes the gradual disintegration of the basement membrane, and ultimately stimulates the ameloblasts on its other side to begin the process of **amelogenesis** – the laying down of enamel matrix.

As the basement membrane disintegrates, the early dentine and enamel layers come into contact with each other, and once this junction is mineralised during the apposition process, it forms the **amelodentinal junction**.

The apposition process is illustrated in Figure 8.2.

As the odontoblasts continue the dentine layering process and move away from the amelodentinal junction, they remain attached to the junctional tissue by developing cellular extensions, which will eventually lie within mineralised tubes of dentine – the **dentinal tubules**. The layer of odontoblast cells themselves will ultimately lie along the outer rim of the pulp.

The ameloblasts will continue the process of enamel mineralisation until the tooth erupts, but are then lost.

Mature enamel and dentine

During the maturation stage of tooth development, ameloblasts actively remove the organic material components of the enamel matrix and replace it with vast amounts of the mineral **calcium hydroxyapatite**. This maturation process occurs from the first formed areas of the tooth – the cusps, incisal edges and occlusal surfaces, and continues towards the outer enamel surface.

Subsequent waves of mineralisation then occur over the surface of these first areas and progress towards the neck of the tooth. Consequently, the cusps, incisal edges and occlusal surfaces are the most mineralised regions of the mature tooth.

Mature enamel forms the hardest tissue in the body, and is composed of crystals of calcium hydroxyapatite laid out in prisms (rods), which run from the amelodentinal junction to the tooth surface over the crown of the tooth. The tissue is 96% inorganic, and has neither vascular nor nerve tissue within it, so once lost, it cannot renew or replace itself.

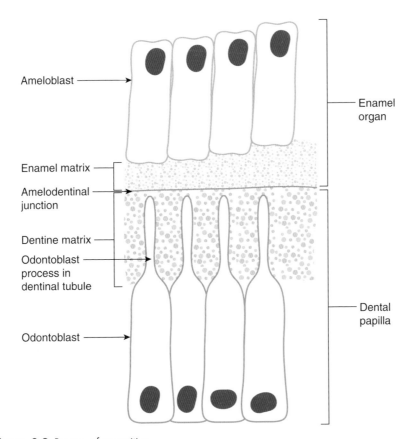

Figure 8.2 Process of apposition.

It forms a translucent covering over the underlying dentine of the tooth, so it is dentine that produces the colour shade of the teeth.

Once erupted into the oral cavity, the enamel can become further mineralised by the uptake of fluoride ions into the hydroxyapatite structure – this is the basis for the prevention of dental caries, by making the enamel surface more resistant to attack by the weak organic acids produced by cariogenic micro-organisms.

The process of caries development and progression through the tooth is well detailed in various dental textbooks, and is summarised here later.

In addition to enamel loss due to caries, the tissue can also be lost in the following ways:

- **Abfraction** – fracture of sections of enamel at the cervical region of the tooth, especially due to parafunctional forces or as occurs to single standing teeth with heavy occlusal loads
- **Abrasion** – loss of cervical enamel due to frictional forces from heavy tooth brushing, especially if combined with the use of gritty toothpastes

TOOTH ANATOMY

- **Attrition** – loss of biting surface enamel due to heavy tooth-to-tooth contact, especially due to bruxing or extensive chewing actions
- **Erosion** – loss of smooth surface enamel due to acid erosion, where the acid has not been produced by micro-organisms

The maturation of dentine follows a similar process to that of enamel, but as stated previously, the odontoblast cells remain within the outer pulp tissue for life. Dentine is therefore able to continue forming within the tooth, and often does so as **secondary dentine**.

Mature dentine is also composed of calcium hydroxyapatite crystals, but is only 70% mineralised. The mineralised tissue develops hollow tubes where the odontoblast extensions lay during early dentinogenesis, and these are present throughout the tissue as hollow dentinal tubules.

The tubules contain tissue fluid and nerve fibrils from the pulp tissue, so that the dentine can detect pain sensation. There are no blood vessels within the dentine, instead the odontoblasts receive nutrients from the tissue fluid.

The mature tooth tissues are illustrated in Figure 8.3.

TOOTH ANATOMY

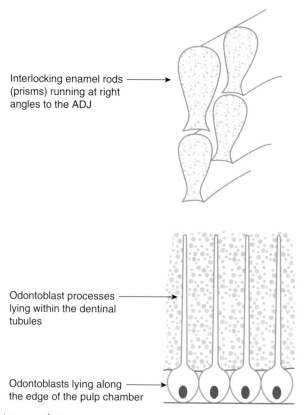

Interlocking enamel rods (prisms) running at right angles to the ADJ

Odontoblast processes lying within the dentinal tubules

Odontoblasts lying along the edge of the pulp chamber

Figure 8.3 Mature tooth tissues.

Root and pulp

The development of the root follows a similar pattern to that of crown formation.

Root development begins once the crown of the tooth is formed, starting at the cervical loop. The formation of Hertwig's root sheath stimulates the inner layer of cells to differentiate into odontoblasts, which then begin laying down early dentine, in a similar manner to the process of dentinogenesis that occurred in the crown.

As the process continues, the root sheath disintegrates and the overlying cells forming the dental sac differentiate into **cementoblasts** and begin laying down a layer of cementum over the developing root.

The contact layer between the early root dentine and the cementum forms the **dentinocemental junction**.

Where multi-rooted teeth are forming (molars and the upper first premolar), the root sheath differentiates into several structures from the original single root trunk.

At the same time as the root and cementum are forming, the inner cells lying at the centre of the dental papilla differentiate into the pulp tissue.

The pulp is the vital tissue of the tooth and has both blood and nerve supplies, which all enter the tooth through the apical foramen.

The pulp chamber within each tooth will be shaped in a similar manner to that tooth, with the pulp in the crown known as the coronal pulp, and that in the root as the radicular pulp. The latter is usually referred to as the 'root canal'.

Some teeth have additional contact between the pulp and the surrounding periodontal ligament via **accessory canals**.

A typical tooth form is illustrated in Figure 8.4.

Dental caries

The process of dental caries begins as an attack on the sound tooth by weak organic acids, produced as by-products by certain oral bacteria as they digest sugars and carbohydrates from foodstuffs.

The most damaging foods are those containing non-milk extrinsic sugars – those added during food manufacture and processing.

The acid production lowers the overall pH of the oral cavity from 7, and once the critical pH of 5.5 is reached, enamel demineralisation occurs and an early carious lesion develops.

Remineralisation of the enamel can occur at this point by the application of topical fluoride to the lesion, but once cavitation has occurred and the amelodentinal junction is breached, only restoration can restore the tooth.

The hollow, tubular nature of dentine allows the caries to progress more rapidly through it than occurs through enamel, and the overlying enamel will

TOOTH ANATOMY

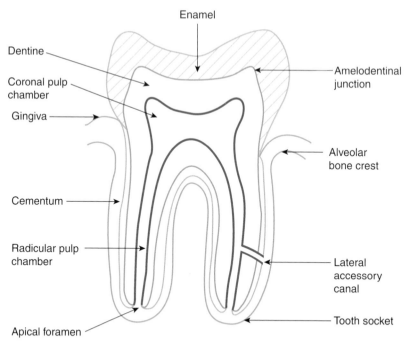

Figure 8.4 Typical form of a tooth.

become undermined. As the carious lesion mushrooms through the dentine structure, the unsupported enamel will fracture away and open the cavity to more attack and destruction. The nerve fibrils within the dentine tubules will be transmitting intermittent pain sensations at this point, particularly when stimulated by temperature changes. This is called **reversible pulpitis**.

As the caries approaches the pulp chamber, the odontoblasts lining it will lay down secondary dentine in an effort to avoid the pulp chamber being breached by the micro-organisms. If unsuccessful, the pulp tissue will become contaminated and eventually die as **irreversible pulpitis** occurs. If untreated, a periapical abscess may develop.

The tooth will now require endodontic treatment to save it, otherwise the source of infection will require removal by the extraction of the tooth.

DENTAL ANATOMICAL NOMENCLATURE

As all dental care professionals know, the tooth surfaces are referred to specifically in relation to their adjacent anatomical structures, depending whether they lie in the maxillary or mandibular dental arch.

The general terminology in use is summarised as follows:

- **Labial** – surface adjacent to the lips, applies in both arches and relates to incisor and canine teeth
- **Buccal** – surface adjacent to the buccinator of the cheeks, applies in both arches and relates to premolars and molars
- **Palatal** – surface adjacent to the palate, applies to all maxillary teeth
- **Lingual** –surface adjacent to the tongue, applies to all mandibular teeth
- **Occlusal** – biting surface of posterior teeth, applies to both arches and relates to premolars and molars
- **Incisal** – biting edge of anterior teeth, applies to both arches and relates to incisors (canines have a cusp rather than an edge)
- **Mesial** – interdental surface of all teeth closest to the midline of each arch
- **Distal** – interdental surface of all teeth furthest from the midline of each arch

These are illustrated in Figure 8.5

TOOTH MORPHOLOGY AND FUNCTION

Each tooth in each dental arch has its own individual shape and size that make them easily recognisable to all members of the dental team. This is called their morphology, and is related to the function of each tooth.

In the primary dentition there are five teeth in each quadrant of the mouth; central and lateral incisors, a canine and first and second molars.

In the secondary dentition there are eight teeth in each quadrant; central and lateral incisors, a canine, first and second premolars and first, second and third molars. The morphology and function of the similar teeth in each dentition is the same.

Features of individual teeth are illustrated in Figure 8.6.

Central incisor

- Chisel-shaped crown with an incisal biting edge
- Single root
- Palatal or lingual surface has a raised area called the **cingulum**
- Upper permanent central incisor is the largest of all incisors
- Lower central incisor is the smallest tooth
- Functions are:
  - To cut into food and separate bite-size chunks from the food product
  - Assist tongue in making certain speech sounds ('th')
  - Assist lips in making certain speech sounds ('f')

TOOTH ANATOMY

TOOTH ANATOMY

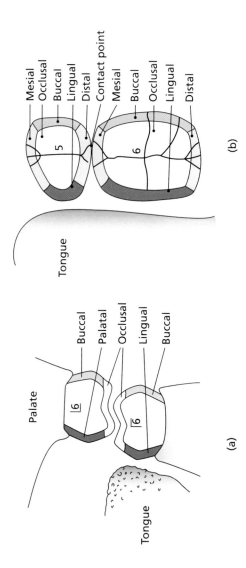

(a)

(b)

Figure 8.5 Tooth surfaces. (a) Surfaces of the teeth – mesial aspect; (b) surfaces of the teeth – occlusal aspect. (From Hollins, C. (2008). *Levison's Textbook for Dental Nurses*, 10th edn. Blackwell Publishing, Oxford. Reproduced with permission from John Wiley & Sons, Ltd.)

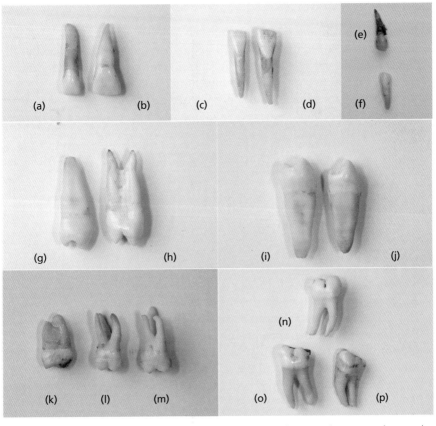

Figure 8.6 Features of individual teeth. (a) Upper right lateral incisor; (b) upper right central incisor; (c) lower left central incisor; (d) lower left lateral incisor; (e) upper right canine with some alveolar bone attached; (f) lower left canine; (g) upper left second premolar; (h) upper left first premolar; (i) lower left second premolar; (j) lower left first premolar; (k) upper right third molar; (l) upper right second molar; (m) upper right first molar; (n) lower right first molar; (o) lower left second molar; (p) lower left third molar.

Lateral incisor

- Narrow, chisel-shaped crown with an incisal biting edge
- Single root
- Lower lateral incisor sometimes has a second (lingual) root canal, especially if the root has bifurcated (split into two)
- Palatal or lingual surface has a cingulum
- Function is to bite in a scissor action with the upper incisors, and break off separate bite-size portions
- Uppers can be congenitally absent, or develop as abnormally small teeth – often called **'peg laterals'**

TOOTH ANATOMY

Canine

- Robust tooth forming the 'corner' of each dental quadrant
- Incisal edge is sloped to a sharp cusp tip that lies more mesially than distally
- Single root, longest of all teeth, bony covering forms the canine eminence of the alveolar process, especially prominent in the maxilla
- Root apex sometimes curves distally slightly
- Upper and lower canines have a cingulum, the upper is joined to the cusp tip by a palatal ridge
- Functions are:
  - Pierce food and tear into it
  - Support the oral soft tissues at the 'corners' of the oral cavity
  - Provide 'guidance' for normal occlusion, especially when the mandible is moved sideways

First premolar

- Not present in primary dentition
- Are the permanent successors to the deciduous first molars
- Has occlusal surface arranged as two cusps lying bucally and palatally, or buccally and lingually (upper or lower)
- Cusps are of equal height in uppers, but lingual is always smaller in lowers
- Mesial and distal edges of all are raised into **marginal ridges**
- Upper has two distinct roots, or a bifurcated root, lying in the same orientation as the cusps
- Root apices sometimes curve distally
- Concavity between the roots mesially is called the **canine fossa**, and can be a harbour for micro-organisms and calculus in patients with periodontal disease
- Lower first premolar has one root
- Functions are:
  - Assist canine to pierce and tear food
  - Assist molars to grind food on their occlusal surface
  - Help maintain the shape of the mouth
- Usual tooth to be extracted for orthodontic reasons

Second premolar

- Not present in primary dentition
- Are the permanent successors to the deciduous second molars
- Has occlusal surface arranged as two cusps, like the first premolars
- Cusps are of equal height in all
- Mesial and distal edges are raised as marginal ridges
- Upper is usually slightly smaller tooth than the first premolar

- Lower is usually slightly larger than the first premolar
- Single root, apex sometimes curves distally
- Root apex of uppers can lie very close to the floor of the maxillary antrum
- Functions as for first premolars
- Lowers are sometimes congenitally absent
- Can become impacted in either arch, following the early loss of their deciduous predecessor and the eruption of the permanent first molars, so that the arch space for the second premolars is lost

First molar

- Primary first molars are succeeded by the first premolars, and are the smaller of the deciduous molars
- Widely divergent roots present in deciduous molars, with the crown of the developing first premolar lying contained by them
- Permanent first molars are the largest of all teeth
- Upper has occlusal surface arranged as four cusps; two buccally and two palatally
- Fifth palatal cusp of uppers may develop as the **'cusp of carabelli'**
- Lower has five cusps; three buccal and two lingual
- Mesial and distal edges are raised as marginal ridges
- Uppers have three roots arranged as a tripod: (1) large palatal, (2) shorter mesiobuccal and (3) distobuccal – apices of latter two are sometimes curved distally
- Lowers have two roots arranged as mesial and distal, apices are sometimes curved distally
- Junction of the roots beneath the crown is called the **furcation area** and can be a harbour for micro-organisms when periodontal disease is present
- Function is to grind and masticate food chunks so that they can be swallowed
- Root apices of uppers can lie close to, or even penetrate, the floor of the maxillary antrum

Second molar

- Primary second molars are succeeded by the second premolars, and are the larger of the deciduous molars
- Widely divergent roots present in deciduous molars, with the crown of the developing second premolar lying contained by them
- Crown of both upper and lower is smaller than that of the first molar
- Has occlusal surface arranged as four cusps
- Mesial and distal edges are raised as marginal ridges
- Uppers have three roots, arranged as for the first molar and sometimes curved distally

- Lower has two roots, arranged as for the first molar and sometimes curved distally
- Furcation area present in both
- Function as for the first molar
- Root apices of the upper can also lie in close proximity to the floor of the maxillary antrum

Third molar

- Not present in the primary dentition
- Not always present in the secondary dentition
- Referred to as **'wisdom teeth'**
- Morphology varies widely
- Smaller crown size than the second molar usually
- Has occlusal surface arranged as three or four cusps, with marginal ridges present
- Uppers usually have three roots, but not always
- Lowers usually have two roots, but not always
- Furcation area present unless the roots are fused together
- Function as for the first and second molars
- Often extracted if involved with recurrent bouts of disease, or if impacted and associated with pericoronitis

A comparison of the primary and secondary dentitions is given in Table 8.1.

Eruption dates of primary teeth

The process of eruption is covered in Chapter 7.

The primary teeth begin forming in the embryo at around the sixth week, always starting in the anterior mandibular region before the anterior maxillary region, and then progressing posteriorly in both arches. This time line is broadly reflected in the eruption dates of the dentition, as shown in Table 8.2.

Eruption dates of secondary teeth

The secondary teeth begin forming in the foetus at around the twelfth week, and follow the same positional progression as the primary dentition. Again, this is broadly reflected in the eruption dates, as shown in Table 8.3.

OCCLUSION

While both the primary and secondary dentition are erupting into the dental arches, the **occlusion** of the individual develops – this is the final contact

Table 8.1 Comparison of primary and secondary teeth.

Feature	Primary	Secondary
Odontogenesis	Around sixth week of embryological development	Around twelfth week of embryological development
Eruption begins	Around 8 months old, with lower central incisors	Around 6 years old, with lower central incisors and first molars
Full set total	20 teeth	32 teeth
Teeth per quadrant	Central and lateral incisor, canine and first and second molar	Central and lateral incisor, canine, first and second premolar and first, second and third molar
Notation	From midline backwards, referred to as A, B, C, D and E in each quadrant	From midline backwards, referred to as 1, 2, 3, 4, 5, 6, 7 and 8 in each quadrant
Crown features	Smaller than secondary, white, thin enamel, large pulp chamber	Larger than primary, yellowish, thicker enamel, relatively smaller pulp chamber
Roots	Same number for all as for secondary, molar roots widely divergent to encompass developing crown of premolars, roots are resorbed before exfoliation	Same number for all as for primary, plus premolars, no divergence, no root resorption unless trauma or pathology present, no exfoliation
Miscellaneous	Rare to be congenitally absent Rare to be impacted	Third molars, upper lateral incisors and second premolars sometimes congenitally absent Impaction common

Table 8.2 Eruption dates of primary teeth.

Tooth	Letter	Uppers (in months after birth)	Lowers (in months after birth)
Central incisor	A	10	8
Lateral incisor	B	11	13
Canine	C	19	20
First molar	D	16	16
Second molar	E	29	27

TOOTH ANATOMY

Table 8.3 Eruption dates of secondary teeth.

Tooth	Number	Uppers (in years after birth)	Lowers (in years after birth)
Central incisor	1	7–8	6–7
Lateral incisor	2	8–9	7–8
Canine	3	10–12	9–10
First premolar	4	9–11	9–11
Second premolar	5	10–11	9–11
First molar	6	6–7	6–7
Second molar	7	12–13	11–12
Third molar	8	18–25	18–25

positions that the teeth in both arches occupy, both within each arch as well as between the two arches.

The final positions of the teeth, especially the secondary dentition, are influenced by other factors:

- **Jaw size** – if one or the other jaw is smaller than required to accommodate the erupting teeth, there will be crowding in that arch, if larger than required the teeth will be spaced
- **Jaw relationship** – if the mandible develops behind its usual position, a Class II occlusal relationship occurs, if ahead of its usual position a Class III occlusal relationship is likely
- **Muscular influences** – these will vary depending on the position of the mandible, as well as naturally, and the obvious one is a tight lower lip musculature, which can trap some incisor teeth and cause their retroclination, or cause them to develop beyond the lip and cause the proclination of the upper incisors
- **Parafunctional habits** – such as thumb or finger sucking, which can cause abnormal muscular forces on the whole of both arches, causing both retroclination of lower incisors and proclination of uppers, as well as buccal cross-bites

Normal occlusion occurs when the upper and lower arches interdigitate correctly, and is referred to as Class I occlusion. The following features are evident:

- Centre lines of both arches are coincident
- Mesiobuccal cusp of the upper first molar lies in the buccal groove of the lower first molar
- Cusp of the upper canine lies in the point between the lower canine and first premolar
- Upper arch is slightly wider than the lower arch, so that the upper buccal cusps lie on the buccal sides of the lower teeth

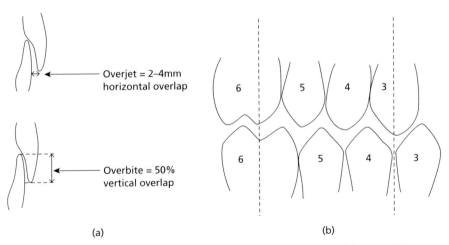

(a)   (b)

Figure 8.7 Class I occlusion. (From Hollins, C. (2008). *Levison's Textbook for Dental Nurses*, 10th edn. Blackwell Publishing, Oxford. Reproduced with permission from John Wiley & Sons, Ltd.)

- Horizontal overlap of the lower incisors by the upper incisors is between 2 and 4 mm – this is the **overjet**
- Vertical overlap of the lower incisors by the upper incisors is 50% - this is the **overbite**

Class I occlusion is illustrated in Figure 8.7.

When the occlusion does not develop correctly, there is a degree of damage possible to individual teeth by the occlusal trauma produced when the arches bite out of synchrony with each other. Some teeth may experience heavy occlusal loading because of this, and may wear more easily, or fracture.

The subjects of occlusion and malocclusion are covered in detail in texts covering orthodontics and prosthodontics.

TOOTH ANATOMY

Chapter 9

Periodontal anatomy

Anatomically, the periodontium is the collective term used for those structures that support the teeth in the jawbone, and traditionally includes the following tissues:

- **Cementum** – hard tissue covering of the root that anchors the periodontal ligament to the tooth
- **Periodontal ligament** – connective tissue attachment between the tooth and the alveolar bone
- **Alveolar bone** – specialised ridge of bone over each jaw, where the teeth sit in their sockets
- **Gingivae** – specialised soft tissue covering of the alveolar processes, that are also in attachment with the teeth at their necks

The gross anatomy of the periodontium in relation to a tooth is illustrated in Figure 9.1.

CEMENTUM – HISTOLOGY

Once the crown of a tooth has developed, during odontogenesis, the formation of the root tissues begins. As root dentine is laid down, the root sheath disintegrates and the cells of the dental sac in immediate contact with the developing dentine differentiate into **cementoblasts**, and begin to lay down cementum.

The initial layer contains no cells, and as it matures it forms the **dentinocemental junction**. Later layers are formed more rapidly and enclose the cells that have formed the tissue in that area – these are then called **cementocytes.**

Mature cementum is around 65% inorganic, with the majority of its crystal structure made up of calcium hydroxyapatite. The crystals lie within a matrix of fibrous tissue, with the ends of collagen fibres from the periodontal ligament inserted into the outer layer of the cementum. These fibrous ends are called **Sharpey's fibres.**

Basic Guide to Anatomy and Physiology for Dental Care Professionals, First Edition. Carole Hollins.
© 2012 John Wiley & Sons, Ltd. Published 2012 by John Wiley & Sons, Ltd.

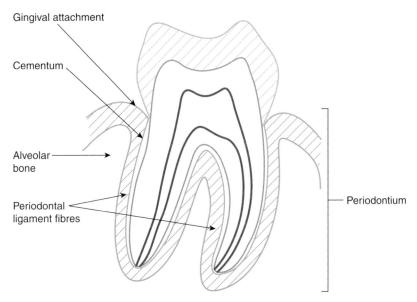

Gingival attachment

Cementum

Alveolar bone

Periodontal ligament fibres

Periodontium

Figure 9.1 Gross anatomy of the periodontium.

Any cementoblasts not enclosed in the matrix are positioned on the outer surface of the cementum, and they can continue laying down more tissue layers when required. As the tissue contains no blood vessels or nerve tissue, nutrients from the periodontal ligament are taken in by this outer ring of cementoblasts.

The microscopic relationship of cementum to the other periodontal tissues is illustrated in Figure 9.2.

PERIODONTAL LIGAMENT – HISTOLOGY

The periodontal ligament forms from the dental sac tissues, as the tooth root and cementum are developing. It is a fibrous connective tissue composed of various cell types suspended in its intercellular matrix. The main cells are **fibroblasts,** which form the **collagen fibres** of the periodontal ligament.

The fibres are not dispersed randomly throughout the matrix, but are ar-ranged as directional bundles that run mainly between the cementum and the alveolar bone of the tooth sockets. Some run between adjacent teeth, while others run into the surrounding gingivae. Where any fibres are attached to cementum or bone, they do so by the specialised Sharpey's fibres at their ends.

The main function of the ligament is to act as a shock absorber for the tooth, and allow it to 'bounce' in its socket during normal occlusal loading and usage. This prevents the tooth from being traumatised by normal actions such as chewing.

PERIODONTAL ANATOMY

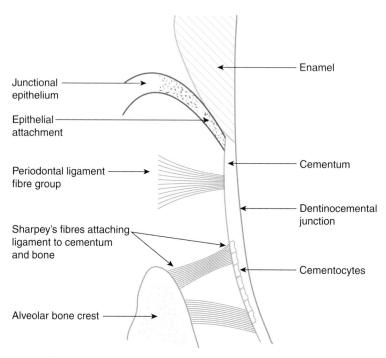

Figure 9.2 Relationship of cementum to periodontium.

The various periodontal ligament fibre groups and their functions are summarised as follows:

- **Alveolar crest fibres** – run from the alveolar bone crest to the cementum at the neck of the tooth; prevent extrusion and intrusion of the tooth, as well as resist tilting and rotation
- **Horizontal fibres** – run horizontally from the alveolar bone to the cementum, just below the crest fibres; resist tilting and rotation of the tooth
- **Oblique fibres** – run at an angle from the alveolar bone down to the cementum; prevent intrusion and rotation of the tooth
- **Apical fibres** – occur at the root apex and run between the bone and cementum; prevent extrusion and rotation of the tooth
- **Transeptal fibres** – run between the cementum of adjacent teeth through the interdental region; maintain the gingival attachments between the teeth and therefore their positions in the dental arch
- **Free gingival fibres** – run from the cervical cementum into the gingival papillae; maintain the gingival cuff around each tooth

The various fibre groups are illustrated in Figure 9.3.

The transeptal fibres are those most important to the success of orthodontic treatment, as sufficient time must be allowed after treatment for the fibres to

PERIODONTAL ANATOMY

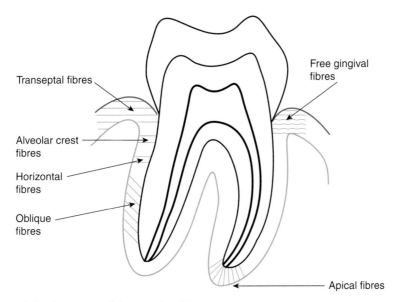

Figure 9.3 Fibre groups of the periodontal ligament.

become stable in their new positions. Use of retainers to hold the re-aligned teeth while these fibres become stable is imperative if the treatment is not to relapse. In most cases, retention should continue for years.

As with most connective tissues, the periodontal ligament contains various cells that can perform different functions, including osteoblasts lining the alveolar bone surface, blood cells and undifferentiated cells that can develop and repair the tissue as necessary. So both the alveolar bone and the cementum of the tooth can repair themselves from the pool of cells within the periodontal ligament tissue.

The ligament is vascularised and provides nutrients for itself and the cementum, and it also has a sensory nerve supply that transmits pressure, pain, touch and temperature changes. The ability of the periodontal ligament to transmit these various sensations, and allow the detection of even the slightest change to the dentition, is called **proprioception**.

Any member of the dental team will be aware of a patient's ability to detect the slightest alteration to their dentition following dental treatment, when a premature contact has been created.

ALVEOLAR BONE – HISTOLOGY

Histologically, the bone of the alveolar processes is very similar to that of the basal bone making up the maxilla and mandible, which in turn is the same as 'ordinary' bone throughout the body. However, alveolar bone only forms in

PERIODONTAL ANATOMY

the presence of tooth germs as the teeth develop, and it resorbs away when the teeth are lost.

Microscopically, the alveolar bone is composed of cells within an inorganic matrix of calcium hydroxyapatite crystals, collagen and intercellular substance. The cells that actually lay down the bone are **osteoblasts,** and as with cementum, some of them become embedded in the bone structure and mature into **osteocytes.**

The osteocytes lie within tubular canals as the calcified matrix is laid down in concentric layers around them. The layers eventually form a structure called a **Haversian system,** which encloses the canal through which blood vessels and nerves run – the **Haversian canal.**

The outer edge of each system is lined by osteoblasts, allowing the tissue to change shape and remodel or repair itself as necessary. During orthodontic treatment, the forced movement of the teeth in a particular direction causes bone resorption on that side of the tooth, and the laying down of new bone on the trailing side of the tooth. In effect, the teeth are dragged through the alveolar bone with a wake of new bone forming behind them.

The histology of bone is illustrated in Figure 9.4.

The outer surface of the bone is covered by a thick connective tissue layer called the **periosteum.** Beneath this is **compact bone,** which is composed of tightly packed Haversian systems with few spaces between, making it very strong. Beneath the compact bone is a more open structure with many spaces between a latticework of bony trabeculae – this is called **cancellous bone,** and is much lighter in weight.

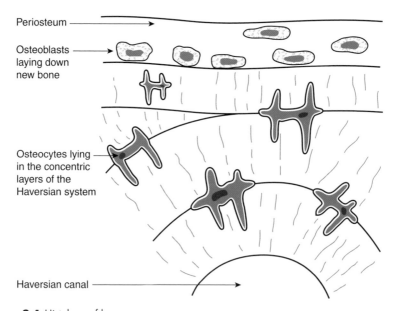

Periosteum

Osteoblasts laying down new bone

Osteocytes lying in the concentric layers of the Haversian system

Haversian canal

Figure 9.4 Histology of bone.

PERIODONTAL ANATOMY

The tooth germs, and therefore their bony sockets, develop in the cancellous bone of the alveolar processes. The sockets are lined by a rim of compact bone called the **lamina dura**, where the Sharpey's fibres of the periodontal ligament are attached. This appears as a distinct white rim around the edges of each tooth socket on a radiograph, and loss of the rim indicates the presence of some form of dental pathology, such as an abscess.

GINGIVAE – HISTOLOGY

The gingivae are the soft tissues that cover the alveolar processes in both jaws. There are three distinct areas of gingival coverage, as follows:

- **Attached gingiva** – that cover the majority of the alveolar process, and that is firmly attached to the underlying bone
- **Marginal gingiva** – that form the gingival margin of the teeth, which is free from the underlying bone and follows the shape of each tooth in the arch, as well as extending between the teeth in the contact areas – the level at which these two areas meet is called the **free gingival groove**
- **Junctional tissues** – the specialised gingival tissue lying within the gingival crevice and forming the anatomical junction between the teeth and the oral epithelium

The attached and marginal gingivae are both forms of **masticatory mucosa,** a type of specialised epithelium found in some areas of the oral cavity. Microscopically, the tissue has the following features:

- **Keratinised surface epithelium** – providing a tough, protective surface to the gingivae, which is able to withstand abrasion from food particles and oral health products
- **Ridged basement membrane** – providing a firm base to the gingivae
- **Thick ridged lamina propria** – firm connective tissue attachment to the alveolar bone, with no elastic fibres or submucosa present – this is the **mucoperiosteum**
- **Free gingival fibres** – of the periodontal ligament run into the marginal gingivae, and maintain their shape around each tooth, also help the lamina propria to produce the stippled appearance of healthy gingivae

JUNCTIONAL TISSUES – HISTOLOGY

These are the specialised tissues that form the **gingival crevice** – the point where the soft tissues of the oral cavity are in direct contact with the hard tissues of the tooth. The area may also be referred to as the **gingival sulcus**.

PERIODONTAL ANATOMY

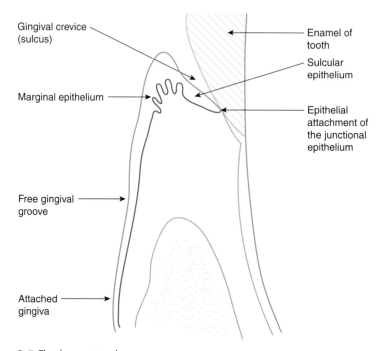

Figure 9.5 The three gingival areas.

It is the point where the integrity of the periodontium has to be maintained in order to avoid the devastation of periodontal disease, and the resultant tooth loss that can occur.

The relationship between the three gingival areas and the tooth is illustrated in Figure 9.5.

The inner surface of the marginal gingiva lies in contact with, but is not attached to, the tooth surface – this is referred to as the **sulcular epithelium**, and the gutter-type space it creates is the **gingival crevice**. This space is usually up to 3 mm in depth in healthy gingivae, and is filled with **gingival fluid**.

Sulcular epithelium is not keratinised, and the basement membrane and lamina propria are not ridged.

Gingival fluid is a watery secretion from the lamina propria of the junctional epithelium cells, and contains antibodies and white blood cells as a defence mechanism against micro-organism attack.

The point at which the soft tissues and the tooth are attached to each other is called the **epithelial attachment**, and is a specialised region of **junctional epithelium**.

Normally, the attachment occurs at the neck of the tooth onto enamel, but it can also exist as an attachment to cementum or dentine.

Microscopically, the cells of the junctional epithelium are packed loosely together, so that the tissue is more permeable to the movement of leucocytes out into the gingival sulcus, to help fight the bacterial plaque biofilm.

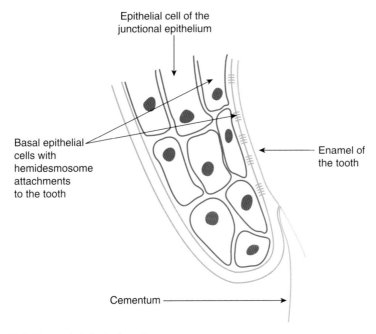

Epithelial cell of the
junctional epithelium

Basal epithelial
cells with
hemidesmosome
attachments
to the tooth

Enamel of
the tooth

Cementum

Figure 9.6 The epithelial attachment.

The basal layer of cells, those that are in contact with the tooth itself, have a mechanical attachment between themselves and the tooth surface, called a **hemidesmosome**. This region forms the **epithelial attachment** of the junctional epithelium to the tooth.

The cells in this region have a rapid turnover, so that a firm mechanical barrier exists between the tooth and the gingivae at all times, except when disease is present.

The epithelial attachment is illustrated in Figure 9.6

PERIODONTIUM AND DISEASE

The increased permeability of the junctional epithelium is a two-way process, and it also allows the invasion of micro-organisms in the bacterial plaque biofilm, and their toxins, into these tissues.

The typical initial inflammatory response that then occurs will present as **gingivitis.**

Initially, the gingivae will swell as the blood supply to the area increases – this swelling forms a **false pocket**, as the gingival sulcus has not deepened.

The increased blood supply to the area will also bring more leucocytes and antitoxins to help fight the bacterial invasion, and will show as bleeding on probing, flossing or tooth brushing. This tends not to occur in smokers, possibly

PERIODONTAL ANATOMY

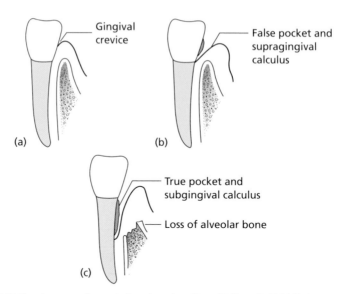

Figure 9.7 Development of a periodontal pocket. (From Hollins, C. (2008). *Levison's Textbook for Dental Nurses*, 10th edn. Blackwell Publishing, Oxford. Reproduced with permission from John Wiley & Sons, Ltd.)

due to the vasoconstrictive effects of some tobacco products. Consequently, the absence of bleeding on probing should not be assumed to indicate a healthy periodontium in these patients.

As the junctional epithelium thins to allow greater permeability still, it is more easily traumatised, and microscopic ulceration will occur. This allows more bacterial and toxin invasion still, and the deeper layers of the tissue will become involved. The bacterial plaque biofilm will become mineralised above the gingivae by the action of saliva, forming **supragingival calculus**.

Once the disease process affects the periodontal ligament, the condition of **periodontitis** is diagnosed. The epithelial attachment is lost, the gingival sulcus deepens beyond 3 mm and a **true periodontal pocket** forms.

This harbours the biofilm and allows the mineralisation of the deeper layers of plaque into calculus by minerals from the gingival fluid, forming **subgingival calculus**. As the disease advances, the alveolar bone will become involved, and the tooth will gradually loosen and become mobile.

In addition, as the leucocytes battle with the invading micro-organisms and each are destroyed, pus will form.

The development of a periodontal pocket is illustrated in Figure 9.7.

Although oral health efforts and maintenance by the dental team and the patient can halt and reverse this process, the re-attachment of the soft tissues to the tooth surface is never as strong as the original epithelial attachment.

PERIODONTAL ANATOMY

Chapter 10

Salivary glands

The salivary glands are present in the oral cavity as either numerous minor glands dotted throughout the oral mucosa, or as one of the three pairs of major salivary glands.

All salivary glands are classed as **exocrine glands** – they produce secretions that are transported to the oral cavity through tube-like structures called **ducts**.

Other structures elsewhere in the body are classed as **endocrine glands** – their secretions pass directly into the adjacent vascular system and are transported distantly by the circulatory system, to their area of action. Examples are certain glands within the pancreas and the stomach.

Both types of glands have their secretions controlled by the effects of motor nerve transmission, via the autonomic nervous system.

MAJOR SALIVARY GLANDS – GROSS ANATOMY

The three pairs of major salivary glands are as follows:

- **Parotid** – located between the ramus of the mandible and the ear, and deep to the muscles in that area
- **Submandibular** – located in the posterior area of the floor of the mouth, beneath the mylohyoid muscle
- **Sublingual** – located in the anterior area of the floor of the mouth, above the mylohyoid muscle

The location of the major glands is shown in Figure 10.1.

The parotid gland secretes saliva into the oral cavity via **Stenson's duct**, which has its opening against the buccal surface of the upper first and second molar teeth, in the cheek.

The submandibular gland secretes saliva into the floor of the mouth via **Wharton's duct**, which opens beneath the tongue, adjacent to the lower incisor teeth.

Basic Guide to Anatomy and Physiology for Dental Care Professionals, First Edition. Carole Hollins.
© 2012 John Wiley & Sons, Ltd. Published 2012 by John Wiley & Sons, Ltd.

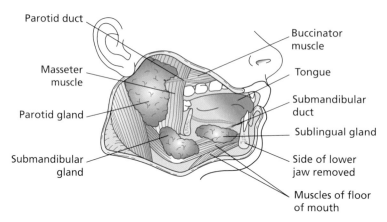

Figure 10.1 Major salivary glands. (From Hollins, C. (2008). *Levison's Textbook for Dental Nurses*, 10th edn. Blackwell Publishing, Oxford. Reproduced with permission from John Wiley & Sons, Ltd.)

The sublingual gland secretes saliva into the floor of the mouth via **Bartholin's duct** in a similar location to Wharton's duct.

As dental care professionals will be aware, these three areas tend to be the main locations for calculus build-up in the patients' mouth.

MAJOR SALIVARY GLANDS – MICROSCOPIC ANATOMY

The three pairs of major salivary glands begin development in the embryo at around the seventh week, as growths of epithelial tissue from the oral ectoderm.

As the epithelial layer folds in on itself and grows into the underlying mesoderm layer, the secretory cells and ducts are formed, which will eventually produce and secrete saliva.

Connective tissue forms around the glands to anchor them to the surrounding anatomical structures, as well as to divide each gland into lobes and lobules, by forming septa. In the parotid and submandibular glands, the outer layer of connective tissue forms a capsule around the whole salivary gland. The vascular and nerve supplies to the glands run in the septal connective tissues.

The inner surface of each duct is lined by specialised epithelial cells called **secretory cells**, which are grouped together at the end of the ducts as **acini** – these resemble a bunch of grapes, and are similar in layout to the microscopic structure of the alveoli in the lungs, as well as to other glandular tissue in the digestive system.

The secretory cells are one of two types in each gland, and the predominant cell present tends to determine the type of saliva produced:

- **Mucous secretory cells** – produce a thick, mucus-like secretion, which aids lubrication in the oral cavity, and contains minerals and enzymes

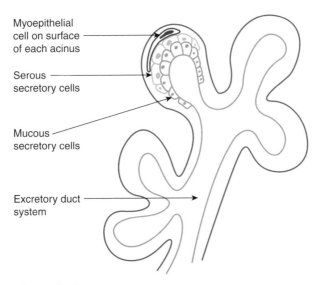

Myoepithelial cell on surface of each acinus

Serous secretory cells

Mucous secretory cells

Excretory duct system

Figure 10.2 Salivary gland acini.

- **Serous secretory cells** – produce a thin, serum-like secretion containing immunoglobulins and electrolytes

In glands that produce both types of saliva rather than one or the other, such as the submandibular glands, both types of secretory cell are present.

Although the secretory cells produce saliva constantly, there are instances where its secretion into the oral cavity needs to be rapid, such as at mealtimes. Specialised contractile cells called **myoepithelial cells** are found on the outer surface of each acinus, and these act to contract and squeeze so that the saliva secretion is forced into the duct and out of the gland more quickly.

The microscopic appearance of the acini is illustrated in Figure 10.2.

Histologically, the minor salivary glands are the same as the major glands, but with much shorter ducts, as they are located in the epithelial layer throughout the whole of the oral mucosa. A special group of them lie at the base of the circumvallate papillae of the tongue, and are called the **von Ebner glands**.

The salivary secretions of all glands are controlled by the autonomic nervous system, which in turn is triggered by a complex sensory receptor system involving taste, smell and the presence of food in the mouth.

Any of these triggers causes an increase in parasympathetic activity to the glands, resulting in an increased blood flow to them as well as an increase in mucous cell secretion of saliva. Sympathetic activity tends to reduce the volume of salivary secretion, leading to a dry mouth.

The drug atropine blocks parasympathetic nerve activity, and can therefore be used in dentistry to reduce salivary flow while patients undergo dental treatment. Use of the drug tends to be limited to maxillofacial surgical sessions, rather than to general practice.

SALIVARY GLANDS

Table 10.1 Salivary gland innervation.

Salivary gland	Cranial nerve	Branch	Saliva type and volume
Parotid	Glossopharyngeal Trigeminal	None Auriculotemporal	Mainly serous Up to 25% volume
Submandibular	Facial	Chorda tympani	Serous and mucoserous Up to 65% volume
Sublingual	Facial	Chorda tympani	Mainly mucous Up to 10% volume
Minor salivary glands	Facial	Greater petrosal	Mainly mucous Less than 5%

All of the salivary glands are innervated by parasympathetic divisions of various cranial nerves, as shown in Table 10.1.

FUNCTIONS OF SALIVA

Although saliva appears as a watery fluid in the mouth, it contains many different components that differ between each salivary gland, depending on the main type of secretory cell present.

It is slightly alkaline, due to its electrolyte components, but maintains the oral cavity at a neutral pH of 7 between meals.

The different components are related to the various functions and roles of saliva, as shown in Table 10.2.

Patients with low mineral content, mainly watery saliva, tend to develop little calculus but have a higher caries incidence than patients with high mineral content saliva.

The latter group tend to have thick, stringy saliva and develop calculus more readily, in the absence of adequate oral hygiene. They also tend to have a lower incidence of caries, often despite inadequate dietary sugar control.

DISORDERS OF THE SALIVARY GLANDS

Xerostomia

This is the uncomfortable condition of a dry mouth due to the decreased production of saliva. The condition is relatively common, and has several causes:

- **Irradiation** – of the head and neck area, usually as radiotherapy treatment for cancer

SALIVARY GLANDS

Table 10.2 Components and functions of saliva.

Component	Function or role
Minerals – sodium, calcium, potassium and their electrolytes – such as phosphates	Neutralise dietary acids Buffering to maintain stable pH in the oral cavity Also allow mineralisation of plaque to form supragingival calculus
Salivary amylase	Digestive enzyme that begins starch digestion, before food is swallowed Also called ptyalin
Secretory IgA	Immunoglobulin (antibody) present to fight infections, such as periodontal disease Promotes wound healing Commonest antibody of the immune system
Leucocytes	White blood cells, as a defence mechanism against oral infection and disease
Mucus	From the mucous secretory cells, to aid lubrication and allow speech and swallowing to occur
Lysozyme	Antibacterial enzyme, to aid in defence of the oral cavity against disease Promotes wound healing
Urea	Metabolic waste product, to be excreted
Water	Carrying agent for other components Aids with lubrication for speech and swallowing Dissolves food particles to allow taste sensation Cleansing action by dislodging food particles from around the teeth

- **Medications** – any that mimic the effects of the sympathetic nervous system, as well as certain drugs such as tricyclic antidepressants
- **Sjogren's syndrome** – a syndrome that occurs in conjunction with an autoimmune disorder, such as rheumatoid arthritis, where the body's defence system attacks itself and destroys its own glandular tissues (such as the salivary glands, and the lacrimal glands in the eye)

As all dental professionals know, saliva has many functions in the oral cavity, and any reduction in its production will have serious oral consequences:

- Increased incidence of dental caries, as the self-cleansing ability is lost
- Increased risk of oral infections, as the defence capability is reduced
- Increased risk of oral soft tissue trauma, as the protective mechanism is reduced
- Problems with speech, swallowing and chewing, as the lubrication effect is reduced

SALIVARY GLANDS

- Poor taste sensation and lack of food enjoyment, as the taste buds cannot function correctly in a dry field

Other than to change any sympathomimetic drugs where possible, there is little else that can be done to ease the condition other than to give salivary stimulants, although research is ongoing into salivary gland tissue transplant too.

Dental patients suffering from the condition should be advised as follows:

- Frequent recall attendance to monitor for the onset of caries and other oral problems
- Use of artificial saliva sprays, or constant water sipping
- High standard of oral hygiene, and especially the use of topical fluoride products to strengthen teeth against caries
- Dietary advice to avoid cariogenic products
- Avoidance of oral health products containing alcohol

Salivary calculi

These are stones, or **sialoliths**, which form in the duct of the gland and obstruct the flow of saliva to the mouth. They occur most frequently in the Wharton's ducts of the submandibular glands, as these are the longest of the ducts and the salivary secretions must travel upwards to reach the oral cavity.

The presence of the chalky stones will cause saliva retention and painful swelling of the gland affected. They can be seen on a suitable radiograph as a radiopaque stone within the duct, or even visibly as a yellowish stone at the duct opening beneath the tongue.

When the submandibular gland is affected, the resultant swelling in the floor of the mouth is called a **ranula**. When one of the minor salivary glands is involved, especially on the lips and due to trauma, the resultant fluid-filled swelling is called a **mucocele**.

Treatment is by surgical removal of the sialolith, or of the salivary gland itself.

Viral infection

The specific viral infection involving the *Paramyxovirus* and its attack on the parotid salivary glands is called **mumps**. It usually occurs in childhood, and can affect one or both of the glands, causing an acute inflammation and swelling with a general feeling of malaise.

Vaccination is available as part of the MMR (measles, mumps and rubella) programme, but the theoretical link of MMR to autism (which has since been disproved) has left some patients unvaccinated. Teenage and young adult males are particularly at risk of the disease affecting the testes, which could lead to infertility in the worst-case scenario.

As with many viral infections, there is no specific treatment available other than to provide symptomatic relief using analgesics

Nicotinic stomatitis

This condition occurs in smokers, and is associated with damage to the hard palate and its associated minor salivary glands by the heat from the cigarette (or pipe or cigar).

The palatal trauma causes hyperkeratinisation and whitening, while the salivary gland ducts are inflamed and appear as red spots over the palatal surface.

Ptyalism

Excessive salivation, or ptyalism, is a symptom associated with an underlying disease rather than a disorder in its own right.

It can occur due to any of the following disorders:

- Periodontal disease
- Oral soft tissue injury, or trauma, including from dental appliances
- Oesophagitis and other conditions causing acid reflux
- Disorders affecting the nervous system, including Parkinson's disease and mercury poisoning

Treatment is focussed on the causative disease and the relief of its symptoms, although some drugs that act on the parasympathetic nervous system may be used to directly reduce the salivary gland secretions too.

SALIVARY GLANDS

Index

Note: Page numbers with italicised f's and t's refer to figures and tables, respectively.

Basic Guide to Anatomy and Physiology for Dental Care Professionals, First Edition. Carole Hollins.
© 2012 John Wiley & Sons, Ltd. Published 2012 by John Wiley & Sons, Ltd.